THIN FROM WITHIN

THE *GO WITH YOUR GUT* WAY TO LOSE WEIGHT

ROBYN YOUKILIS

Photography by
ELLEN SILVERMAN

KYLE BOOKS

This book is dedicated to my generous tush—thank you for being my eternal teacher on the road to loving myself exactly as I am.

Published in 2018 by Kyle Books
www.kylebooks.com

Distributed by National Book Network
4501 Forbes Blvd, Suite 200,
Lanham, MD 20706
Phone: (800) 462-6420
Fax: (800) 338-4550
customercare@nbnbooks.com

10 9 8 7 6 5 4 3 2 1

ISBN 978-1-909487-75-8

Project Editor: Christopher Steighner
Copy Editor: Ivy McFadden
Designer: Nicky Collings
Photographer: Ellen Silverman
Food Stylists: Kate Schmidt,
    Nora Singley
Prop Stylist: Kaitlyn Duross Walker
Production: Nic Jones, Gemma John,
    and Lisa Pinnell

Library of Congress Control Number:
    2017958931

Color reproduction by ALTA London
Printed and bound in China by C&C
    Offset Printing Co., Ltd.

Important Note:
The information and advice contained in this book are intended as a general guide to healthy eating and are not specific to individuals or their particular circumstances. Many substances, whether sold as foods or as medicines and used externally or internally, can cause an allergic reaction in some people. Neither the author nor the publishers can be held responsible for claims arising from the inappropriate use of any remedy, weight loss, or healing regime. Do not attempt self-diagnosis or self-treatment for serious or long-term conditions before consulting a medical professional. Do not undertake any self-treatment while taking other prescribed drugs or receiving therapy without first seeking professional guidance. Always seek medical advice if any symptoms persist.

CONTENTS

FOREWORD

Robin Berzin, M.D.

For a long time our definition of health has pivoted on the external. How we look gets more airtime than how we feel. And yet we know that when it comes to the myriad of chronic conditions so many of us battle in the modern age—from weight gain to uncomfortable digestive issues, chronic fatigue to hormonal imbalances and more—it is truly what is on the inside that counts.

In the past few years new research has shed light on how gut health defines overall health. We know that the microbiome—the trillions of bacteria that live inside our bodies—not only help to digest our food but also impact countless other functions.

We know that different bacteria populations are associated with weight gain versus weight loss and that the health of your microbiome can dictate how fast your metabolism runs, how often you get sick, and even how happy (or sad) you regularly feel.

Yes, the medications we take and the foods we eat define the composition of these populations. But beyond that, we now have proof that certain lifestyle factors—including environmental toxins, stressors, hydration, and activity level—can affect not only how our gut behaves and how we digest our food, but also which bacteria in our systems live and die.

All of this together is what is known as the science of "systems biology"—the idea that the body is an interconnected matrix, constantly in flux in response to stimuli from both inside and outside. The systems biology approach helps us understand why "eat this, not that" and calorie counting regimens don't work—our bodies are much more complicated, and much more intelligent, than that.

Still with all this groundbreaking research, the key question is, how do we take what the science is telling us and make it relevant to our daily lives. In my 10-plus years as a physician working on the cutting edge of medicine, what I've seen missing—and the reason why so many people are still struggling with stubborn weight and gut issues—is a truly inside-to-outside perspective that makes sense with a fast-paced, modern lifestyle.

This is what makes *Thin from Within* special. In this book, Robyn Youkilis has taken her experience with the hundreds of people she has coached one on one and married it with the latest science. She's created a step-by-step food and life plan for shedding weight and finding optimal health by focusing first on your insides—your gut.

This approach is the only one I see sustainably work for people.

Let Robyn guide you to achieving your personal goals and beyond in her caring and thoughtful way. Be patient and go at your own speed. And as you'll learn in this book, listen to your gut. Remember, the key to success is truly already within you.

INTRODUCTION

I've struggled with my weight for most of my life. I've had good days and bad days completely based on how tight my jeans felt when I pulled them on. Despite being a best-selling author; appearing as a wellness expert on national television shows like *The View*; helping hundreds of clients through my health coaching practice, Your Healthiest You; and reaching even more on social media—I'm just like millions of other women out there who look in the mirror and think, "That tush is too much!"

Everyone has her their own journey, their quest to feeling vibrant and happy in their body. For me, it began when, in a desperate attempt to lose weight, I finally stopped eating junky diet foods and started eating real foods and focusing on truly nourishing my gut.

I'm now at my lightest weight and the most comfortable I've ever been in my body, well into my thirties, even after having a baby. But it wasn't that long ago that I was totally frustrated with doing "all the right things" without seeing the right results.

I know I'm not alone. The average adult gains about one pound of weight each year from age twenty-five on. This fact, along with a slowing metabolism, increased stress levels, and a whole host of other reasons leads to why we find ourselves with weight to lose at some point in our adult lives. But, as easy as it is to pack on pounds, you can instead choose to listen to your body, drop the distracting mental chatter, and optimize your digestion. This is the your gut's secret to finding your best body no matter what stage you're at in your life.

I hear success stories all the time from my inspiring clients and friends who have followed my approach to gut health and weight loss. Women from Brooklyn to LA, Australia to the UK tell me my approach has helped them understand their bodies and feel good after a lifetime of diet drama and belly woes. In my first book, *Go with Your Gut,* I explained digestive health in a way that allowed readers to connect with their own gut instincts, learn how to make food choices from a place of inner wisdom, banish bloat, and leverage the amazing power of the simple act of chewing. I have women all over the world making more home-cooked meals, slowing down and discovering the foods and practices that help them feel their best.

Here are just a few stories from my readers and clients:

> With Robyn's help, I learned how to listen to my body by thinking about what kind of food would feel good rather than running on autopilot. While I used to make the same breakfast every day, I began to check in: Did I want one egg or two? Gluten-free toast or leftover roasted vegetables? Did I even need coffee? Did I want some avocado, and how much? I also started prepping food for my day, to ensure I would have good things to turn to rather than the vending machine or an open bag of chips. I no longer feel guilt about food or think about specific foods as being "bad" or "good." Instead, I eat what my body wants and needs, as well as what I know will make me feel like my best self in the long run. — AMY

> I'm now eating breakfast, drinking tons of infused water, loving my gut-friendly smoothies, and actually enjoying cauliflower! Robyn was right—good digestion is the key to everything! Better skin, mental clarity, and more! Thanks for teaching me how to take better care of myself! — PRISHA

Participating in Robyn's virtual Chewing Challenge has taught me to stop inhaling my food and slow down during meals. Now that I chew my food completely not only do I enjoy eating even more, I've realized that I actually don't need as much food as I thought I did! As a result my belly has become tighter, I feel so much more comfortable in my clothes, and I'm loving the pure joy of not having to constantly adjust my pants over my bloated belly! — ALEXANDRA

One of my clients even bragged to me that her husband now eats sauerkraut and kale. That's what I consider real success!

While these transformations illustrate what's possible for anyone with a little information and motivation, what I heard more and more from my readers, clients, and community was the need for a plan; specifically, a weight loss plan.

WHAT THIS BOOK IS ABOUT

This book will show you how stubborn weight can melt away when you tune in to your gut and learn to heal from the inside out. Beyond that, it will show you how to feel comfortable, confident, and energized in this home that is your body.

What I see out in the holistic health world is a lot of dancing around the topic of weight loss. I see a lot of quick-fix approaches that address the symptoms (i.e., belly bloat and weight gain) but not the underlying issues. What's missing is an understanding of why it's so hard to lose the weight and keep it off.

Lucky for you, this book is not another diet book. I won't be assigning grapefruit-only days or cheat days. I'm here to give you straight health talk as someone who is truly passionate about wellness and has spent her life studying health and nutrition. After decades of self-study and an official health coaching certification from the Institute for Integrative Nutrition, I started my coaching practice, Your Healthiest You, almost a decade ago. In my life, I've worn a lot of hats and a lot of clothing sizes, too—probably just like you.

MY DEFINITION OF WEIGHT

Let's first talk about weight and what it really means. Weight is more than just a number on the scale. Even though I only weigh about 10 pounds less than I did ten years ago, I look a hundred times better now. That's because ten years ago, I was carrying around a considerable amount of "emotional weight":

♦ I was desperately searching for how to "get it right" with my food.

♦ I was partying way too much and looking for love in all the wrong places—from the newest leader of the band in the world's skinniest jeans to celebrities who were up to no good.

♦ I was unfulfilled and unhappy in my jobs.

♦ I felt lost in what I was doing with my life and was too afraid to show up when I had glimpses of a "higher calling."

♦ I had no flow or rhythm in my day.

♦ I was carrying credit card debt and quickly depleting the savings I had worked so hard to build.

So what do I mean by "weight" (and weight loss) in the context of this book?

Weight is a feeling in your body...

> A DESIRE TO LOSE WEIGHT IS A SIGN THAT WE WANT SOMETHING TO BE DIFFERENT IN OUR BODIES, BUT EVEN MORE SO, IN OUR LIVES.

For example:

Are you feeling guilty about your food choices, mainly because you think you should "know better"?

Does the anxiety from your high-pressure job show up as daily indigestion or heartburn?

Do you rely on your glass of wine at the end of the day to unwind?

Do you giggle at the idea of "eating your feelings," but know this is exactly what you're doing with your nightly snacking ritual?

Do you feel like you never have enough (in the bank, in your closet, in your pantry)?

Are you feeling unsettled in your life, even though you can't put your finger on exactly what needs to shift?

What you need is a physical weight loss plan, in addition to a plan that will help you shed emotional weight. You've gotta learn to let go of what's not serving you, so you can live your healthiest life and feel amazing.

If your goal is to be lighter in body, belly, and spirit, then this book will guide you there. When I eat according to the Go with Your Gut weight Loss Formula, I feel nourished and full. I'm not worried about calories, and my clothes fit just fine. When I don't eat this way, my digestion tanks (hello, bloating and bad poops), and the old restrictive Robyn diet brain of "eat this, don't eat that" rears its ugly head.

For example, I was on vacation with my family in upstate New York and I forgot my sauerkraut (OMG! How COULD I?). I wasn't making my famous yogurt power parfaits for breakfast. I wasn't structuring my plates like I teach in this book. This was fine for a day or two, but by the fourth day my husband had to literally rip the third serving of Carvel ice cream cake out of my hands.

I share this story to highlight how what you eat affects the delicate balance of bacteria in your digestive tract. When the bacteria in your gut is off kilter, you start to crave more sweets, and you feel exhausted and down on yourself. You can't make solid choices from this place.

The weight loss philosophy I teach in this book is simple and easy to follow. Your body wants you to feel good, and the best way to reach your natural weight is to keep your gut flora happy and balance the other parts of life that "weigh" you down. Together, these two forces will have you looking and feeling fabulous.

WHAT MOST DIETS ARE MISSING

Have you been on a diet, for like, ever, but still have "those last X pounds" to lose? Do you feel like you stay on top of all the wellness trends, but there's still something you're missing . . . a secret trick that everyone knows except you? Or does it feel like you're doing all the right things, but your body isn't responding? Why can't you just lose the weight?

✦ Your gut's not working.

When I say "gut" here, I mean both your physical gut and your gut instincts, your intuition. If your gut isn't working, nothing works. The weight stays on your belly and hips like that annoying ex-boyfriend you can't stop thinking about, but it goes beyond that. You feel stuck in your life. You're doing okay, but you feel like you're not really nailing it—your diet, your workout plan, heck, even what you chose to wear today. After reading this book and following the Go with Your Gut Weight Loss Formula, everything will start to click.

✦ The way you digest your food is the way you "digest" your life.

We'll cover emotional weight loss along with the physical and practical components to powerfully move you forward to your ultimate vision of you. If you've been on the weight loss train for years (or decades), you've probably noticed that even though you've lost weight in the past, it likely didn't feel (or look) the way you hoped it would. It's only when you're willing to look at all the parts of you—body, mind, and heart—that you will finally feel that lightness you've been looking for on the scale.

THE GUT HEALTH–WEIGHT LOSS CONNECTION

When it comes to physical gut health, you may be wondering what exactly digestion has to do with weight loss. "Robyn, I get that gut health may help with annoying issues like bloating and gas, but how does that relate to that extra weight I can't seem to lose?"

The answer is: *everything.*

Yes, healing your gut can help you get rid of embarrassing digestive issues, but it can do so much more than that. There are three main reasons why gut health is directly linked to reaching your ideal weight:

 A healthy gut better absorbs nutrients from the food you are eating.

A healthy gut knows exactly what you need to feel your best. It's your connection to your intuition, your unique gift that directs your best choices in this life.

A healthy gut means a happier you. This is the brain-gut connection I can't wait to share more about.

I'll break down the science and key components of "how" and "why" behind these points in chapter one.

REBECCA'S STORY

My client Rebecca shifted so much more than just her weight using the same principles I'm teaching in this book. When she came to me, she was a busy executive at a big tech company in San Francisco, stressed out and burnt out from eating the "right" foods in the wrong way.

Rebecca was already having salads for lunch and going to the gym regularly when she came to me, but her life and body still weren't clicking. Working in tech, she had way too many options at lunchtime, with a lavish spread of delicious, free food always available. Rebecca followed the Go with Your Gut Weight Loss Formula and learned to actually breathe and chew her food.

Rebecca started using my simple 123 Food Freedom Tool (which you'll learn on page 67!) at lunchtime in the crazy cafeteria. She would go to the bathroom before hitting the cafeteria and simply stand in the stall for a few deep breaths, one hand on her heart and one on her belly. She'd ask herself what she really wanted to eat and what would feel great. By plugging this tool into her routine, she started making simple,

nourishing choices that follow the Good Gut Rule of Five (see page 26 if you want to take a peek). Rather than stressing over food decisions like she used to, it started to feel easy to choose the option she knew was best for her.

Rebecca also began cooking for herself more. As a single gal with a full-time job, the meal prep tips were "life-changing". When she stocked her fridge and pantry the Go with Your Gut way, she stopped reaching for the office dark chocolate almonds every afternoon and stopped ordering takeout every night. Get this: Rebecca used to travel internationally for work eight or more times a year, and she would bring her own meals while flying business class! Keeping her digestion regular by bringing her own food on the road was key to her transformation.

Since restoring her gut through cooking, chewing, and breathing, Rebecca feels relaxed, light, and free around food. She recently switched jobs to a company more aligned with her lifestyle, is studying to become a health coach, and started teaching yoga classes. How cool is that?! Wondering how you can make some of the shifts Rebecca made? Well . . .

WHAT YOU'LL LEARN IN THIS BOOK

In this book I'll teach you my simple GO WITH YOUR GUT WEIGHT LOSS FORMULA: a revolutionary approach to lose weight, heal your gut, and freakin' love your body and life. You'll drop pounds and the mental chatter that weighs on your heart, keeps you feeling stuck, and makes you feel less than fabulous in your body.

You'll learn to listen to that little intuitive voice inside that knows exactly what you need to eat, how you need to move, and how you need to live your life—even if you suspect you've been ignoring it.

You'll get all the information and inspiration you need to lose weight and get your digestion going, but you'll also feel amped to sparkle up your career, relationships, and spirituality—because all areas of your life are connected.

Best of all, you'll find a sense of ease. There will be less of the distracting "should I, shouldn't I" drama in your head. You will feel grounded, supported, and clear on what choices are best for your body and for your life. You will be thin from within.

Ready to get started?
Let's do this.

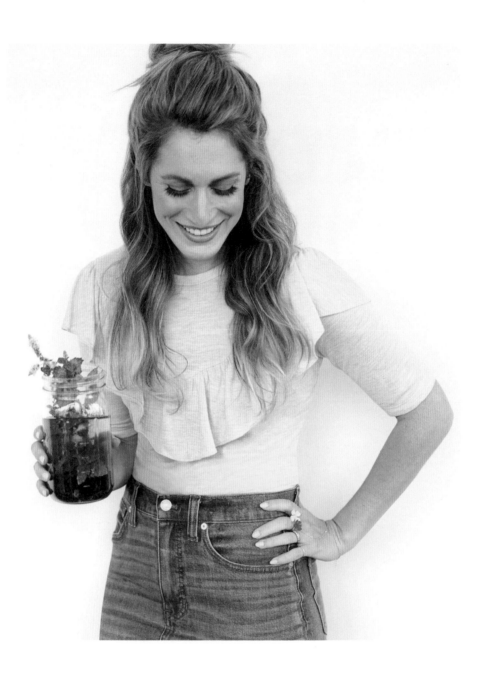

chapter one

CONFESSIONS OF A SERIAL DIETER

So many women I talk to are dealing with most (or all) of these symptoms . . .

- ◆ Inability to lose weight and keep it off

- ◆ Uncomfortable bloating and puffiness

- ◆ Constipation and/or diarrhea

- ◆ Feeling tired, even after eight hours of sleep

- ◆ Dull skin and/or embarrassing acne

- ◆ Stress and anxiety that never seem to go away

- ◆ Trouble falling or staying asleep

And a lot of these women are drinking green juice and going to Pilates on the weekends.

If you picked up this book, you have weight loss goals, but likely you are experiencing some of these other symptoms, too. At this point I'm sure you're frustrated with two-week cleanses and strict meal delivery plans because they don't fit into your life long-term.

I'M JUST LIKE YOU

It can be easy (and delicious!) to lose weight and feel incredible in your body, but I didn't always know that. Just a few years ago, I was exactly where you are, with so many weight loss and lifestyle tools swimming around in my head that I felt like I didn't know where to start.

I tried everything—the 3-Day Diet, the Cabbage Soup Diet, Weight Watchers, the 21 Day Fix, and more—to muscle my body into a weight I deemed was acceptable for my height and frame. I tried to exist on minimal calories to "get back on track" post-vacation. I bought supplements that promised to boost my metabolism and help me shed pounds effortlessly. I was looking for everything outside of me to "fix" me.

MY HISTORY OF DIETING

Growing up, my mom cooked nourishing, real food 90 percent of the time, so I developed a deep love of food and eating. I mean, who wouldn't, when you were served gourmet dishes like coq au vin and lemon meringue pie on the regular? The problem started when I began picking up messages from TV shows and commercials, in magazines, and from the other girls at junior high that I needed to be on someone else's plan to be happy. So I'd stick to sandwiches on whole wheat, carrot or celery sticks, and anything 100 calories or less in a tiny package. I'd be famished by the end of the day and dig into the cabinets for cookies, chips, and anything chewy and sweet I could get my hands on. I could eat Fig Newtons for days and days.

The first real diet I remember going on was the 3-Day Diet, a low-calorie plan of hot dogs and cottage cheese that's supposed to trigger quick weight loss. My mom would do it every other month or so to slim down, and one month I decided to join her. I think I lost two pounds, which I immediately gained back when I returned to my "normal" way of eating.

My obsession with losing weight and wanting to feel great in my body continued into my twenties, as I tried to find myself and figure out what course my life was taking.

I was always trying to eat the most food for the least amount of calories. I loved eating, just like my dad, and I never wanted to feel deprived or like I was eating tiny portions. I would load up on things like low-fat popcorn and baked potato chips . . . stuff you can eat cups on cups of for about 50 calories. The problem? I never felt physically satiated because there's not a ton of real nutrition in those foods.

I didn't understand how to properly feed myself because I was so disconnected from my body.

WHAT SHIFTED THINGS FOR ME

You might be thinking . . .

Okay, so how did you do it, Robyn? How did you finally lose weight and turn your story into your life's work without it all feeling so hard?

Well, it starts with a love story. This may sound like I'm about to share a story of falling in love with a person, but it's even deeper, bigger, and better. This is about falling in love with my life. It does start with a special person, though . . .

When my husband, Scott, and I first started dating, shopping at the farmers' market and cooking was a way for us to connect. I dropped the packaged food and picked up the best of the best. I noticed that the more "real" foods I ate, the less I craved the My Little Pony fruit snacks and the less I was turning to food for comfort.

I was starting to feel better in my body, but it wasn't just about eating healthier food—it was about the time I spent in the kitchen. While I was cooking, I wasn't trying to "fix" anything. I felt creative and inspired. Cooking was my first meditation practice. It was a way for me to slow down and be in the moment. This newfound sense of being present was revolutionary for me.

Cooking was not only the first step in my body and diet transformation, it was the catalyst for a new career that lit me up.

Once I got cooking, I couldn't stop talking about the yummy foods I was creating on the regular. My friends could tell how passionate I was about food and nutrition, and one of them suggested that I check out the Institute for Integrative Nutrition (IIN), the world's largest health coach–training program. One week later, I enrolled.

I was terrified to take so big of a leap, but every fiber in my body, my gut, was telling me yes.

I WAS STILL OVEREATING AND OVER-SNACKING AT NIGHT. HEALTHY HAD ALMOST BECOME ANOTHER DIET FOR ME, AND IT STILL FELT LIKE MY BODY WAS SOMETHING I WAS TRYING TO FIX.

Shortly after graduating from IIN, I built a successful coaching practice on how to fit healthy eating and cooking into their busy lives. I had finally found my path. I was doing something that I was jazzed about, and a layer of what I refer to as "emotional weight" was being shed.

I was definitely healthier, but still struggling with my physical weight. I felt 10 to 15 pounds heavier than I knew my body wanted to be; my outsides weren't matching my insides.

HOW THIS ALL BECAME NEXT LEVEL

My biggest shift in body, weight, and mind happened when I focused on nourishing my gut and taking care of myself from the inside out. When my husband and I began talking about starting a family, I shifted my focus from "How skinny can I be?" to "How can I create the most ideal 'home' for my future baby to live in?" And then I had an aha moment: Our bodies are our homes—this is where we live. Shouldn't we treat them right?

I let go of trying to look a certain way. I slowed down even more at mealtimes and chewed my food completely. I began to focus on the foods (and the activities) that made me feel my best. And guess what? The foods that made me feel (and eventually look) my best were those deeply nourishing foods, the foods that feed and balance the microbiome (aka your gut).

WHY THE GUT?

Your gut is the center of your being—it digests and assimilates nutrients from the food that you eat. It's where the majority of your immune system resides, and it also plays an important role in your mood and hormones. If I wanted to build the best home possible, it made sense that my gut was the place to start. The more I dove into the gut-health world, the more I saw that healing the gut would resolve so many of my clients' issues (even the most stubborn ones). By focusing on healing the gut, these women were able to calm their digestive issues and also calm their out-of-control emotional eating.

As I mentioned at the beginning of this book, there are three main reasons why gut health is directly linked to reaching your ideal weight:

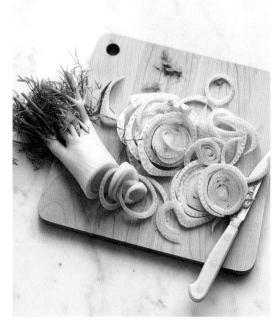

 A healthy gut better absorbs nutrients from the food you are eating

 A healthy gut knows exactly what you need to feel your best

 A healthy gut means a happier you

1 A HEALTHY GUT BETTER ABSORBS NUTRIENTS FROM THE FOOD YOU ARE EATING

Contrary to much diet advice out there, it's not just what you eat or the number of calories you consume, but how your body is using those calories. Your digestive system's main jobs are both to break down the food you eat and to absorb and assimilate the nutrients from that food.

You might be eating nutritious, whole foods most of the time, but still feel foggy, uninspired, and generally "less than" your brightest self. Why? Because if your gut isn't in tip-top shape, it's not properly absorbing all the vitamins and nutrients from your food, which means your cells don't have the fuel they need to do their jobs. It's like having a jewelry box full of diamonds, but not having the key to unlock the box to wear those beautiful gems.

Your body may also enter starvation mode, known in scientific circles as metabolic adaptation, where it conserves and stores energy by holding on to fat. This also happens on low-calorie plans. If your body isn't getting enough nutrients, the brain's hypothalamus and pituitary glands work with other endocrine glands to retain calories (i.e., conserve resources) so that your body systems keep functioning.

When your digestion is functioning optimally, your gut absorbs the nutrients it needs from the healthy food you are eating and then signals to your brain that you are satisfied. You won't enter starvation mode because you aren't starving for nutrients. Your body won't need to store excess fat for energy because it trusts that it will get the nutrients it needs when it needs them.

With a healthy gut, you naturally eat a little less (because you are getting more out of what you are eating), dropping those stubborn extra pounds while maintaining optimal energy levels.

YOUR BODY WON'T NEED TO STORE EXCESS FAT FOR ENERGY BECAUSE IT TRUSTS THAT IT WILL GET THE NUTRIENTS IT NEEDS WHEN IT NEEDS THEM.

2 A HEALTHY GUT KNOWS EXACTLY WHAT YOU NEED TO FEEL YOUR BEST

Most weight loss plans don't work because we ignore our bodies in favor of the latest trend. When our gut instinct pops up and says, "Hell no," we ignore it because the louder voice is telling us these stories:

♦ My best friend, Jess, lost 10 pounds doing Whole30 so I should start that plan this week.

♦ All the wellness girls on Instagram are eating gallons of organic almond butter, raw chocolate, and, like, 10 bananas a day—I guess that means I can, too!

♦ Heidi Klum drinks a shot of apple cider vinegar before each meal. ON IT.

When you learn to listen to your unique body, it will lead you to exactly the foods, workouts, and life choices that are best for you in each moment. This isn't something a diet will accomplish for you. You must go deeper and connect to your intuition.

What I found to be the key missing piece during my years of dieting—and the reason I could not lose weight for most of my life—was self-trust. I didn't trust my body one bit. When I craved and ate pizza, I suffered from self-judgment and felt gross. When I ate salad, at first I would feel good for making the "right choice," but I was hungry after and would often end up snacking into oblivion, defeating any of the benefits of eating the salad.

I didn't trust my gut and the signals it was giving me. I wasn't listening.

After years of berating my thighs for not being thin enough and constantly comparing myself to other (smaller, better, more successful, blah blah blah) women, I'm so relieved to be at peace in my body and life, and I want you to feel that way too.

Our bodies are designed to seek optimum health. Your body is on your side and wants you to feel good. When you give it a chance, it will tell you exactly what it needs. This is the more figurative or spiritual part of gut health—it's about reconnecting with your intuition and reconditioning yourself to trust it.

 ## A HEALTHY GUT MEANS A HAPPIER YOU

Many experts refer to the gut as your "second brain" because it contains millions of neurons, which are quite sensitive to emotion. Multiple scientific studies have proven that our brain and gut are connected by an extensive network of neurons, chemicals, and hormones that constantly provide feedback about how hungry we are, whether or not we're experiencing stress, sadness, or even anger. These emotions can trigger a reaction in your gut.

Have you ever felt your belly flip after receiving an e-mail you were dreading? That's the brain-gut connection in action. This is meant to work in our favor: just thinking of what you are going to eat for lunch can release digestive juices and prepare your body to eat before you take your first bite.

The gut-brain connection is a two-way street. Tummy troubles can impact your mood and happiness. Do you know what serotonin is? It's your body's "feel good" neurotransmitter, which means it carries signals along and between your nerves. Serotonin is responsible for regulating a number of body processes, such as sleep and digestion, but its main role is to regulate anxiety, happiness, and mood. In fact, low levels of serotonin have been associated with depression. It's estimated that 90 percent of your serotonin is made in your digestive tract, and that the production of this chemical is reliant on healthy gut bacteria.

If your gut is a mess from poor food choices, stress, and other factors, you're never going to feel the way you imagine your "goal weight" to feel. In other words, even if you reach your weight goal on the scale, without a healthy gut, you may still feel bloated, unsettled, and uncomfortable in your body. If you have a history of dieting (and self-doubt) like me, there's a good chance your gut bacteria is way off, and this is what's stopping you from feeling and looking the way you want.

WHAT IS THE MICROBIOME AND WHY IS IT IMPORTANT?

The microbiome is all the tiny microbes that live in and on our bodies. These little bugs mainly help with digestion and fighting infection, but they also play a role in our moods and happiness levels.

Your microbiome begins to develop at birth. Babies get covered in microbes as they pass through the birth canal, and receive more via their mother's milk. The microbiome continues to grow and change as a result of familial, dietary, and environmental factors.

So, what does the microbiome do? All these little guys help to extract vitamins and other nutrients from the foods we eat and deliver it to all your cells. You can think about your microbiome each time you eat kale and quinoa, as it helps get all the goodness out of these foods and into your body. It's also an essential component to immune function. Seventy to eighty percent of your immune tissues are located within your digestive system. The gut is often the first entry point for pathogens, so keeping it healthy is what helps you avoid illness.

THIS GOES DEEP

When I finally focused on nourishing my gut with both the foods and the mindful eating practices I teach in this book, my physical body started to look the way I had always imagined it in my mind. I lost those stubborn pounds, but, more important, I got off the diet rollercoaster and finally felt at home in my body.

Yes, this is deep, and yes, this whole gut health–weight loss connection is more complicated than just taking a probiotic pill and munching on some greens. Don't worry, though—I'm going to give you a formula for your new way of eating and living, and a manageable plan that you can put in place tomorrow, or even today. But first, we need to get clear on where you are starting from and what your specific goals are. In the next chapter, I'll walk you through just that.

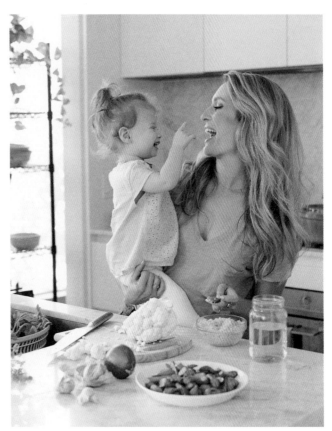

START WHERE YOU ARE

YOU DESERVE TO FEEL AMAZING IN YOUR BODY— INSIDE AND OUT. YOU CAN BE A SPIRITUAL PERSON AND STILL WANT TO LOSE WEIGHT.

If you're hesitant to say you wish your dress size were smaller, you can let out a sigh of relief because here's the truth: You can love and appreciate your body as it is right now and still want to lose weight. Your body is your business, and if you want to look and/or feel different and that desire comes from you—not from the media, your mom, or your boyfriend—it's all right to take action to make your dream body your real body.

Your body and your soul work in tandem, and the better you take care of your physical body, the more able you are to take care of your spirit.

Yes, there are a lot of things that are more important than how much you weigh. In fact, almost everything is more important than how much you weigh.

Now that we've got that out of the way, let's get to work! In this moment, how good do you feel in your body on a scale of 1 to 10? If that number is less than a 9 or 10, you're in the right place. Make a mental note of your number as a way to get honest with yourself and start making loving, gradual changes from this point on so you can feel happy in your body, calm around food, and inspired in your life.

Whenever I get started with new clients, I always use the first session for us to get clear on where they currently are and where they want to be. If you don't know where you want to be, how will you know once you've gotten there?

I created a special workbook to support the practices that I'm teaching you in this book. This will give you a place to get clear on your goals, track your progress and put what you're learning into real action. Head to robynyoukilis.com/books to download your free copy!

A NOTE ON DIGESTIVE DISORDERS

The tips and recipes in this book will help virtually anyone improve their gut health, but there are a few more serious digestive disorders that require particular attention. I've summarized them below. If you think you may have one of these conditions, please talk to your health-care practitioner before undertaking any new plan or supplement regime.

Leaky gut, also known as intestinal permeability, occurs when particles are able to "leak" from your intestine into your bloodstream. This causes inflammation throughout your body, leading to a variety of issues such as food sensitivities, autoimmune diseases, malabsorption of nutrients, skin conditions (like acne and psoriasis), and mood issues.

Crohn's disease and ulcerative colitis are both major categories of inflammatory bowel diseases (IBD). Crohn's disease is a chronic inflammatory condition of the gastrointestinal tract. Ulcerative colitis is a chronic inflammatory condition limited to the colon, otherwise known as the large intestine. Both Crohn's and ulcerative colitis have similar symptoms such as diarrhea, urgent need to move bowels, abdominal cramps and pain, and sensation of not being able to get it all out when you go to the bathroom. General symptoms associated with IBD include loss of appetite, weight loss, fatigue, night sweats, and loss of a normal menstrual cycle.

Small Intestinal bacterial overgrowth, commonly known as SIBO, is when there is excessive bacteria in the small intestine. When in proper balance, the bacteria in the colon help digest foods and assist the body in absorbing essential nutrients. However, when this bacteria invades and takes over the small intestine, it can lead to poor nutrient absorption and digestive discomfort, and may even lead to damage of the stomach lining. Symptoms include nausea, bloating, gas, diarrhea, malnutrition, joint pain, fatigue, skin rashes, eczema, asthma, and even depression. If you have SIBO, you likely need a very different diet than the one offered in this book, so I recommend sticking with the emotional teaching components and guidelines on "how" to eat rather than focusing on the specific foods themselves.

Celiac disease, an autoimmune disease that can occur in genetically predisposed people, is an allergy to gluten that leads to damage in the intestines. When people with celiac disease eat gluten, their bodies mount an immune response that attacks the small intestine, specifically the villi, which are small fingerlike projections that line the small intestine and help with nutrient absorption. When the villi get damaged, nutrients cannot be properly absorbed into the bloodstream. The symptoms of celiac disease can vary greatly and are different in children and adults. The most common signs for adults are diarrhea, fatigue, and weight loss; other symptoms not directly related to the digestive system include anemia, mouth ulcers, headaches and fatigue, joint pain, itchy skin, loss of bone density, and nervous system issues such as problems with balance or numbness in the hands and feet.

DEFYING OLD STORIES

Being a wellness babe is not about being the same size as when you were 24. Getting stuck in that used-to-be mind-set keeps you frustrated no matter how much progress you've made.

When my client Sandy came to me, she couldn't believe what she saw in the mirror. She had always been naturally skinny and was not used to seeing curves on her body. Sandy was so stuck on how she used to look that she felt crappy no matter how many positive shifts she made in her life (or pounds she lost).

Before we started working together, Sandy was lucky if she pooped once a week (she thought this was normal). She had no idea what kale, kombucha, or sauerkraut were, and her family was not on board with her healthy lifestyle goals. Together we did the practical work, but we also did the inner, emotional work. We looked at the things that were weighing on Sandy, more than just a few extra pounds around her hips—what I refer to as "emotional weight."

Now she has a garden where she grows all sorts of vegetables (including kale!) and makes her own sauerkraut. Her sixteen-year-old daughter regularly asks for the recipes from my first book, *Go with Your Gut,* for dinner, and they go to the gym together once a week. She poops daily, and has a lot of good gut tools at hand for when it feels like her life and body aren't flowing.

She's also much nicer to herself. She makes breakfast most days, she's investing in herself both personally and professionally, and she speaks more kindly to herself. She's crafting her self-acceptance, while still continuing to move forward with her body and life goals.

Does she still have days when she looks in the mirror and her thoughts start to drift to a negative place? Sure, but she's making progress every day and learning to trust herself more and more. Instead of focusing on how she used to be, she's envisioning and blossoming into a current and future life that's brighter, expansive, and more beautiful than what's past.

YOUR PERSONAL GOALS

Pull out your new downloaded workbook or cute journal and jot down three specific goals you have for yourself and your health. Sure, weight loss can be one of them, but I encourage you to focus on other positive changes you want to see in your life. Feel free to flip back through the client stories I've shared so far for some inspiration.

GIVE YOURSELF A VISUAL

As we get started, I'm going to make one small request: Take a photo of yourself right now at the beginning of this journey. Why a photo? As humans, we're wired to see our weak spots, the places where we're vulnerable or need improvement. This is why when you look in the mirror, all you see is what you wish were different, even if your bestie says you look amazing. I suggest taking photos because you can't always trust you'll see positive change in the moment. It's not to bash yourself, it's just a check-in to see exactly where you are now. Notice how you look physically, but also energetically and emotionally. You may want to take a moment with your workbook or journal and write down what's coming up for you.

Then set a reminder on your calendar for one month and three months from the date of your initial photo. Use these photos to see how far you've come. Heads up—taking photos of yourself can bring up lots of emotions.

Share your experience in our private Thin From Within Book Club Facebook group—we're here to support one another.

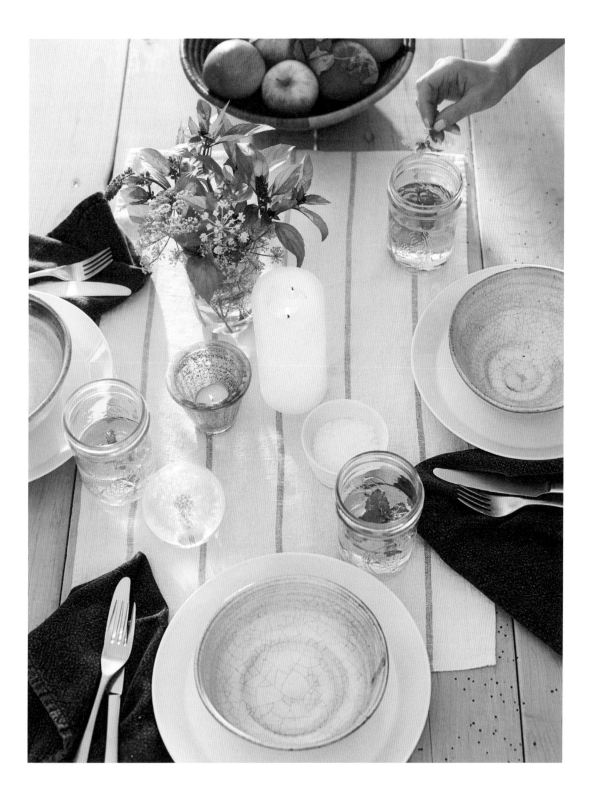

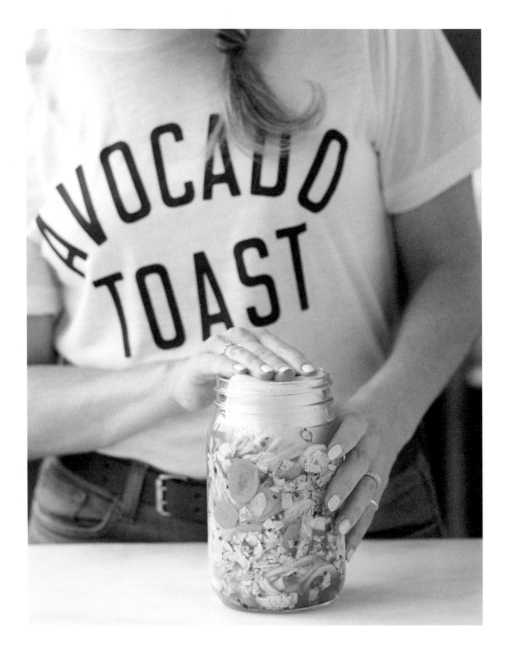

chapter two

THE GO WITH YOUR GUT FORMULA

THE GO WITH YOUR GUT WEIGHT LOSS FORMULA

The Go with Your Gut Weight Loss Formula is life-changing, and revolutionary if you're a recovering dieter like me. You may have picked up this book for the recipes, and even if you only make the recipes and do nothing else, you'll see a huge transformation in your body and life. Cooking changes everything, which is why this book is so recipe-focused.

However, if you want to be like Amy, who lost 6 pounds and, more important, let go of her guilt around eating and food, keep reading. Spend some time with the next few chapters to up level everything you are doing in the kitchen.

My approach to weight loss is based on gut health and smart cooking as well as simple daily practices that shift your mindset and energy. GO WITH YOUR GUT is a four-part formula with the most important practices to incorporate into your everyday life. You can implement these practices whether you cook your meals at home, eat on the road, or somewhere in between. GO WITH YOUR GUT is a food and lifestyle framework to ultimately make your own.

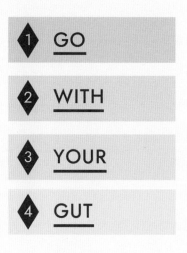

1 **GO**

2 **WITH**

3 **YOUR**

4 **GUT**

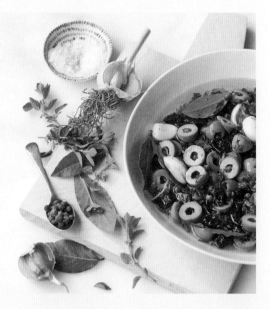

STEP 1

GO

We're going to get right into real talk, because that's who I am and that's what's worked for hundreds of my clients. You need to be **GO**-ing first thing in the morning—and yes, I mean pooping.

You want to have a nice smooth movement— well-formed and easy to pass—first thing in the morning. I know it's not the cutest thing to talk about, but you and I both know how amazing a good poop feels. There's a reason for that! You're not only flushing toxins and waste out of your body, but you feel lighter too.

So how can you make sure you're pooping every day? The first step is to drink a big glass of water as soon as you wake up. I keep an extra-large mason jar filled with filtered water on my nightstand and drink it down as soon as I open my eyes and sit up.

You can step it up by drinking warm or hot water with lemon, but the most important thing is that you're just getting water of some sort down the hatch, and a good amount of it—at least 12 ounces, and as much as 32.

Ready to bump it up a notch further? Try my Go with Your Gut Shot first thing in the morning to get things moving: Simply combine 1 to 2 ounces pure aloe vera juice, ½ ounce raw apple cider vinegar, and a squeeze of lemon juice and shoot it down just like you'd take a shot of tequila with your girls on a Saturday night.

WATER, WATER EVERYWHERE!

Drinking plenty of quality water is essential for good health and weight loss. Here are a few of my top tips about your new favorite beverage du jour from my first book, Go with Your Gut:

♦ Don't drink water with meals. It will dilute your gastric juices. Aim to finish any beverages 30 minutes before each meal and wait an hour after each meal before drinking more.

♦ Avoid adding ice to your water—it puts out your belly's "fire." Your digestive system does better with room temperature or warm water.

♦ Make sure you are drinking enough water each day. Here is a good formula to calculate how much you need: Divide your body weight by two and this is the number of ounces you want to drink each day.

♦ I recommend investing in a home filtration system of some kind and drinking out of glass containers whenever possible (for my favorite water bottles and filters, head to robynyoukilis.com/books).

STEP 2

WITH

Simplify your food **WITH** the Good Gut Rule of Five. I created the Good Gut Rule of Five to show you exactly what to put on your plate at lunch and dinner.

Eating in this way will ensure that you are getting a balance of both macro- and micronutrients, as well as my favorite gut-healing superfoods.

Aim to include one ingredient from each of the five categories that follow for a complete and balanced meal.

MACRO- AND MICRONUTRIENTS

Macronutrients are the caloric components of our foods that most of us are familiar with: carbohydrates, fats, and proteins. Micronutrients are the vitamins, minerals, trace elements, phytochemicals, and antioxidants within our foods that are essential for proper cellular function and good health. Many processed and packaged foods contain plenty of calories, but are lacking in micronutrients (which is why you can seem to eat and eat and eat these foods without being really "full"). I created the Good Gut Rule of Five as an easy way to ensure you're getting a healthy balance of both macro- and micronutrients in the majority of your meals.

◆1 GREENS

Kale, collards, arugula, spinach, lettuce . . . I love 'em all. Aim to have at least two or three big handfuls of greens with most meals. Greens do it all when it comes to gut health and weight loss: They are packed with fiber, which helps fill you up and keep you regular. Plus, leafy green veggies are some of the most nutrient-dense foods, and when you are filling your cells with nutrients (I mean real nutrition, not just calories!), you have more energy and fewer cravings.

◆2 HEALTHY FAT

Avocado, olive and flax oils, almonds, butter from grass-fed cows (so the cows have healthy guts too!), and coconut oil all count here. Add 1 to 2 tablespoons of oil, 1 to 2 ounces of nuts, or ¼ to ½ of an avocado at each meal for a good dose of flavor and satiation. Plus, fats are essential for proper absorption of most vitamins and minerals. I used to be terrified of fats, but now I include them at every meal and am lighter than I've ever been.

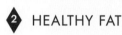

◆3 PROTEIN

Wild salmon, grass-fed beef, organic chicken, tempeh, sprouted lentils, and canned wild sardines are some examples of great go-to protein options on the Go with Your Gut Weight Loss Plan. Protein keeps you full and stabilizes your blood sugar, so you won't keep dipping into your raw chocolate stash or crash halfway through your afternoon meetings.

◆4 FERMENTED FOOD

Including fermented foods on your plate is the good gut secret to weight loss through a healthy microbiome (you need all that great bacteria throughout the day to keep your digestion humming!). Examples include raw sauerkraut, fermented beets, fermented carrots or radishes, and kimchi. Try adding 1 to 3 tablespoons at each meal, and feel free to work your way up to ½ cup or more. If you're not used to the flavor of fermented veggies, try mixing them with avocado to mellow the flavor.

Ideally you should have a fermented veggie with your meal, but if not, you can get your daily dose of probiotics from kombucha, kefir, yogurt, or any of the other sweeter fermented foods.

◆5 COOKED VEGETABLES

Having a cooked veggie or two with my meal (in addition to greens) always makes the meal feel more grounding and filling. Roasted zucchini, broccoli, sweet potatoes, squash, and carrots are all examples of delicious cooked veggies, but this can really be any veggie. I try to roast a bunch of seasonal veggies at least once or twice per week so I always have some cooked veggies on hand and ready to go. If you're on the run, many takeout spots and fancy restaurants have awesome veggie choices these days.

Keep your meals simple and nourishing with these five components.

◆@ *Whether you're making a recipe from this book, or compiling a plate from your local salad bar, I want to see your Good Gut Rule of Five meals! Snap a photo and post to Instagram, Facebook, or Twitter— make sure to tag #thinfromwithin and @RobynYoukilis so I can see your delicious photos and be inspired!*

WHAT ABOUT BREAKFAST?

The recipes in this book will cover you for breakfast—whether you're having a Power Parfait, a gut-friendly smoothie, or a savory option, you'll likely be hitting on many of the Rule of Five categories without even thinking about it! I've found that this rule is most applicable (and most helpful) for the other meals of the day, where we tend to get more confused as to what exactly belongs on our plate.

STEP ◆3

YOUR

Take **YOUR** time for you before everyone else in the space between your day and your evening. This is where things get messy for most of us, even after eating a solid lunch and maybe even making it to that after-work spin class.

When you're finished with your work for the day, take a moment to come back into your body. This step is key in breaking up with mindless eating habits that often greet us at the door.

tip

Are you a stay-at-home mom or at-home anything? You can practice this, too. Go for a walk, lock yourself in your laundry room, lay down on the ground—do something to mark the transition from work to home (even if the physical transition doesn't exist).

If your home space allows you to have a few calm minutes, you can do this as soon as you get home. If everything is in your face all at once as soon as you walk in the door, you might need to sit in your car or find a park bench where you can have a few minutes. Put your phone down—you can check it later. This is your moment to check in with your body and brain and recalibrate. Take a few deep breaths, drop your shoulders, and make yourself a cup of tea or drink a big glass of water if you can. Come back into yourself—acknowledge what happened during your day, and then set an intention for the evening. Are you going to cook yourself dinner? Do some light yoga? Call your mom? What do you want your evening to look (and feel) like?

This moment of recalibration and connection with self is what sets you up for real and sustainable weight loss success—it's essential in closing the gap between how you want to spend your evening and the post-work autopilot that happens for so many of us.

STEP ◆4
GUT

Finally, and probably most important, nourish your **GUT**. You want to be adding extra key nutrients and supplements to love your gut up. Yes, you want to be eating the food from this book first and foremost, but you'll probably need to start taking some probiotics (or remember to take them) and adding in a little extra fiber.

One important tip about probiotics—I recommend taking them at night. This is when your digestive system is at its most relaxed state and your body can assimilate them best. Your organs, digestive system included, rest and repair while you're sleeping. Give your body time to digest your food at night by having an earlier dinner (ideally 3 to 4 hours before bed) so you have space to process your food and the events of your day before you go to sleep.

The last piece of the Go with Your Gut Weight Loss Formula, and one of my own personal weight loss secret weapons, are my Good Gut Gellies (page 165). Add my Good Gut Gellies as a little treat after dinner to get extra fiber in, which is key for a good poop (which brings us full circle back to the first step of my Go with Your Gut Weight Loss Formula: Make sure you GO!).

I'll talk more about probiotics and other key gut supplements on page 58.

The rest of the book builds on the Go with Your Gut Weight Loss Formula. We're starting with "go," aka your morning, in the next chapter. So let's go!

WHAT ARE PRO- AND PREBIOTICS ANYWAY?

Probiotics are the good bacteria your gut needs to carry out digestion properly. Probiotics are found naturally in fermented foods like sauerkraut, kimchi, yogurt, miso, tempeh, and more. The two primary organisms or strains of bacteria in probiotics are *Lactobacillus* and *Bifidobacterium*. We need both to properly break down and absorb our food so we can keep our metabolism humming fast and lose (or maintain) weight.

Prebiotics are nondigestible fibers that promote the growth of beneficial microorganisms in your intestines. Examples include apples, garlic, jicama, dandelion greens, and onions. Think of them as a natural fertilizer that feeds your internal garden.

If you've had tummy troubles for years, the solution isn't to throw as many probiotics and prebiotics at it as you can. They might make you feel worse or keep you stuck to your toilet for days. Do your research or work one-on-one with someone who can help you safely integrate these nutrients into your diet.

A note about antibiotics: Antibiotics kill off bacteria—the bad and the good—so they can cause damage to your gut. If you absolutely must take them, be sure to take a probiotic supplement and eat plenty of probiotic-rich foods during your course of antibiotics to help restore the good bacteria in your gut.

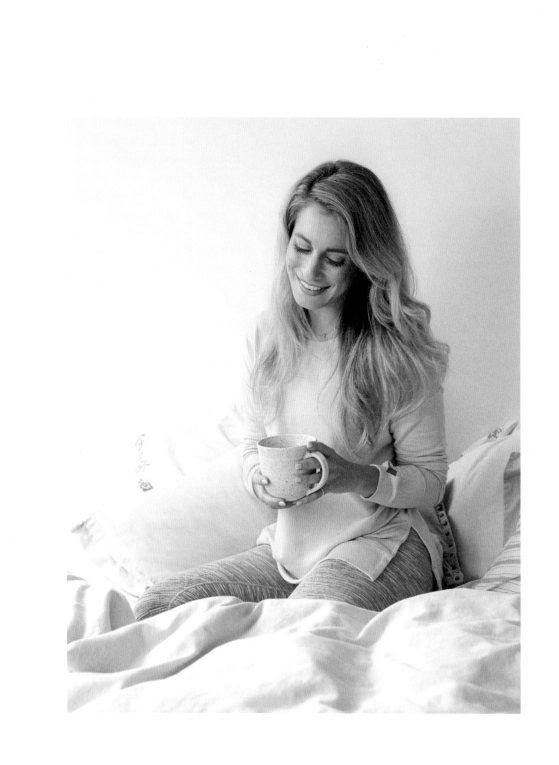

chapter three

YOUR
MORNING
ROUTINE

As I sat up in my bed and took a little stretch, the sunshine beamed in on my face and I could hear the birds chirping outside my window. I thought to myself, "Hello, beautiful day!" I made my way over to my meditation cushion and settled in for my Zen morning routine.

And then I woke up.

My morning reality actually looks more like this: My beautiful daughter is hungry and needs to be changed and fed immediately. My husband—the same. Just kidding! But he does have questions about our dinner plans that night, and my phone is pinging me with email and after email.

Morning "routine"? Most days, it's a challenge just to find a moment to poop in peace.

WHY YOU MIGHT NOT BE GOING NUMBER 2

Maybe you have your own version of my morning reality. I find the reason most of us are not going is because we aren't giving ourselves a moment to come into self at the beginning of the day. All the foods and recipes in this book will help you have nice, easy poops on the regular, but you also need to give your body the time and space to actually go.

When you anchor yourself in your body for a few minutes each morning, not only do you set yourself up for a good poop, but you set the tone for the rest of your day. You are in the driver's seat of your life. Once you are present in your body, you are more likely to make choices that will support yourself all day.

If you're like me and you have a young child or another circumstance that leaves you rolling your eyes at any type of morning routine, I'm not going to ask you to spend hours journaling or chanting on your yoga mat to reap the benefits of a little morning time. Even a smidge counts.

MY MORNING MINUTE

Here's what I do most days: When I wake up, I place one hand on my heart and one hand on my belly and take a few deep breaths. I say some version of the following to myself (think *Goodnight Moon,* but the morning self-care edition) . . .

"Hi, I'm awake. How lovely is that? Good morning body, good morning heart. I've got you. I'm here, this is me. These are my arms, this is my skin, this is my chest, this is my face, I've got you."

When I take that moment to check in with myself, to start the day with ease and calm, not only am I more likely to feel grounded and happy, I'm also much more likely to make positive choices throughout my day.

This minute of calm is what I call my Morning Minute. It's a moment for me to connect with my mind and my body, to get my feet under me before the day gets ahead of me.

There's no one "right" way to do your Morning Minute. Try out a few of the ideas below to figure out what feels best for you.

Yours may be:

♦ 1 minute of breathing deeply into your belly

♦ listening to a short guided meditation

♦ shaking your body out to your favorite song

♦ writing in a journal

♦ reading a snippet from an inspirational book

♦ sipping a cup of tea alone

♦ gently tapping on your body to increase blood flow (or any light movement)

Why is it so important to take this time to chill out? Science shows that mindfulness and meditation lead to decreased levels of stress hormones like cortisol. One study in particular from Georgetown University's Medical Center showed that an eight-week course of daily mindfulness classes lowered inflammatory molecules and stress hormones by around 15 percent. When stress hormones are high, they send messages to your body to store calories as fat, making it harder to lose weight—even if you're eating all the healthy stuff. No joke! High levels of stress hormones can also cause inflammation and other health issues that can keep you from feeling your best.

In addition, you cannot properly digest and absorb the nutrients from your food if you're stressed. Your nervous system exists in one of two states: the sympathetic nervous system (the fight-or-flight response that accompanies stress) or the parasympathetic nervous system. Your parasympathetic system controls homeostasis, your body's sense of balance, and its ability to carry out digestion.

If your sympathetic nervous system is engaged too often, your digestion is impaired because the body is designed to use energy first for survival—it doesn't know the difference between an angry e-mail from your boss or your jumping out of the way of New York's worst cabdriver. If you're stressed, your body puts up the same defenses and dedicates all energy to staying alive, leaving secondary processes like digestion weakened.

When you use your breath and take mini breaks, like my Morning Minute, to de-stress and get your body into the parasympathetic state, your digestive system can do its job. Added bonus: You're also more likely to make decisions from a calm and clear place.

HOW TO PRACTICE DEEP-BELLY BREATHING

Deep-belly breathing is an easy and effective tool for weight loss and improved digestion. And yes, one minute of breathing can absolutely change the course of your day.

- ♦ Start by setting a timer for one minute.
- ♦ Put one hand on your chest and one on your belly.
- ♦ Now breathe deeply into your stomach, letting it get as big as possible on the inhale, then relax on the exhale.
- ♦ Repeat continuously, inhaling and exhaling in this manner, until the timer goes off.

It's really important to let your belly expand fully. We spend so much of our day sucking it in, and that suppresses digestion.

MISSED YOUR MORNING MINUTE?

Ideally you take your Morning Minute at the very start of the day, before it's time to be a mom, a busy executive, a student, or [insert all the other hats you might wear daily]. But if you missed it, you have the power to hit reset and connect with how you want to feel in any moment. Even one minute can make all the difference.

Here are six practical ways you can hit refresh on your day:

1 On your next visit to the bathroom, add in one minute of deep-belly breathing.

2 Go to lunch with a coworker and practice the art of listening.

3 Call a friend just to say "How are you?"

4 Go for a quick walk around the block on your lunch break . . . and leave your phone at your desk.

5 Listen to a song that soothes you or moves you. Bonus points for dancing along.

6 Write down five things you're grateful for.

You can sprinkle these little check-ins throughout your day to feel more calm, focused, and at peace with what is. When you're in that state, you'll feel ready to tackle your big goals while appreciating exactly where you are today.

MAKE IT HAPPEN

Now, what do you need to do to make sure this practice actually happens? Do you need to download a meditation app, set your alarm for 15 minutes earlier than usual, or tell your partner about your new routine?

Think about how you'll make it happen. Consider anything else that needs to shift that you'll want to plan or prepare for.

 Head over to the Thin From Within Book Club Facebook group to share your Morning Minute or if you want more inspiration!

BREAKFAST IS SERVED

The first meal of the day can be a meditative check-in in and of itself, and feel just as awesome as your Morning Minute. Breakfast is an important part of my approach because in all my years of coaching, I've found that my clients are so much less likely to binge later in the day if they've had a balanced breakfast (i.e., something more than a green juice or bagel with coffee). When we deprive our bodies of nutrients, they overcompensate (overeat) when we finally do feed them.

Despite the fact that we know we should eat breakfast, so many women still struggle with this meal or skip it because they just can't deal.

For years, I loved the time I spent in the morning making myself breakfast (remember what I said about cooking being my first meditation? It still is a grounding practice for me). I loved making beautiful, Instagram-worthy plates like perfect scrambled eggs piled high with spicy arugula, fermented hot sauce, and sourdough toast. I was fortunate to have a job and a life that allowed, and actually encouraged, me to take this time each day.

I love this meal now, but everything changed when I got pregnant, and then again when I had my daughter, Navy.

During pregnancy, I couldn't even stomach the thought of eggs or greens. And spending any time over the stove? No thank you.

My cravings changed, my body changed, my life changed. And so my breakfast had to change, too.

I needed a new breakfast—something that would fuel my morning, that I loved eating, and that I could make ahead of time or quickly on the spot when I didn't have time to prep. After much experimentation, the Power Parfait was born. It's basically an upgraded yogurt, fruit, and granola bowl, and was the recipe that triggered my easy post-baby weight loss.

Why? Because I listened to what my gut needed. Instead of trying to force myself to eat something that I thought was the "healthiest" option based on what I had read (and even loved), I listened to my body and what it needed, something I'll be teaching you how to do for yourself in the chapters to come.

The other important "it" factor of this breakfast? It created consistency in my days when, as a new mom, my mornings were anything but.

I created this recipe for me, but I quickly saw how it solved the breakfast conundrum for so many of my clients because it meets the following criteria:

◆ You can prepare a fleet of Power Parfaits all at once, setting yourself up for an entire week . . .

◆ But you don't have to do anything in advance— this breakfast can just as easily come together on the spot!

◆ It contains gut-friendly fiber, probiotics, and prebiotics.

◆ It's packed with protein, which will keep you full for hours.

◆ It's freakin' delicious.

◆ And bonus: Little ones love it, too.

One client wrote to me to say, "I've been making Power Parfaits on Sunday night. This has made the difference between my eating a healthy breakfast and grabbing something fast like a sugary muffin, or worse, skipping it."

note

The Power Parfait, like a smoothie, is a perfect vehicle for superfoods (check out page 59). You don't have to miss out on the fun superfood craze just because you don't drink a smoothie for breakfast or have a super-duper blender!

This breakfast has the power to set your mornings free, whether you're a new mom or just in need of an easy, gut-friendly meal to start to your day.

The following recipe makes one serving— if you're packing up a week's worth, simply line up your to-go containers and measure the ingredients into each one. Feel free to switch up the fruit!

◇

POWER

PARFAIT

BLUEPRINT

Here's the basic formula I use when making my Power Parfait bowls. Each day is a little different because I like to switch up the fruit and granola, but the formula remains the same. For more fun variations and how you can mix up your parfaits, head to pages 82–83.

¾ cup yogurt

¼ cup plain oats

1 teaspoon chia seeds

Small scoop of protein powder

   (check out my faves at robynyoukilis.com/ books)

Splash or two of homemade nut milk or water

¾ cup fresh berries or other chopped fruit

¼ cup low-sugar granola

1 Mix the first five ingredients together.

2 Top with the fruit and granola. Eat immediately or store in the fridge for later!

yogurt

Goat's milk is my favorite, but you can also use organic cow's milk, sheep's milk, or plain coconut milk or nut-based milk yogurt.

oats

Oats are rich in prebiotic fiber and make this bowl so much more satisfying than your average yogurt cup. You can skip this add-in if you're paleo or grain-free.

chia

Chia seeds are rich in fiber and help clean out your digestive tract. Chia seeds are also full of omega-3 fatty acids, which help fight internal inflammation and fuel your brain to produce more feel-good hormones like serotonin.

tip

GRAIN-FREE? USE A COMBINATION OF UNSWEETENED SHREDDED COCONUT AND SLIVERED ALMONDS IN PLACE OF THE OATS AND GRANOLA (OR USE A GRAIN-FREE GRANOLA).

If you're looking for one place to start on your gut health and weight loss journey, start with your morning.

Your breakfast and morning routine set the tone for the rest of the day. This could be the difference between feeling good about your body and great about your life, or feeling like nothing is working out. It's always worth the one extra minute of breathing, or those 10 extra minutes of breakfast prep on the weekend. When my mornings start the way I want them to, I feel like I'm riding with the rest of my day, instead of being pulled along.

note

If your gut is saying HELL NO . . . and you instinctively know that yogurt or a cold and sweet breakfast is not for you, go with your gut, my friend! If you're not really sure what is best for you, experiment! There are plenty of other gut-friendly breakfasts in this book—head to page 75 for more delicious options.

@ *Do you love your Power Parfait as much as I do? Take a photo of your favorite variation and post it to social media— make sure to tag me @RobynYoukilis and #thinfromwithin so I can see your beautiful creations!*

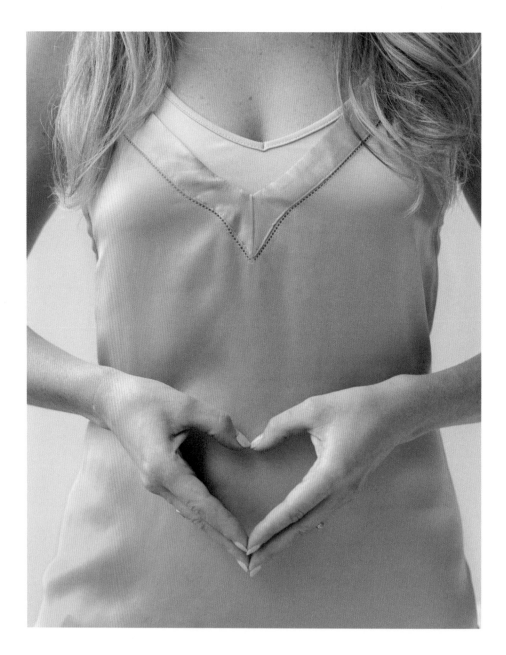

chapter four

THE 3-DAY GOOD GUT RESET

Let's recap what we've covered so far. We got crystal clear on your body image (on a scale of 1 to 10) and your current personal goals. I shared my Go with Your Gut Weight Loss Formula (which you can apply no matter what you have going on) and we did a morning makeover. Fun!

Now it's time to get into the program. In this chapter I'm sharing my 3-Day Good Gut Reset. It's a meal plan designed to jumpstart weight loss and give you a taste for how to structure your meals in a waist-friendly way, every day. Think of this as the starter program for you and your body to become familiar with new foods and methods of eating. To make life easy, I'm providing you with a shopping list and step-by-step instructions so all you have to do is shop and show up!

Can just three days of practice really make a difference? Yes it can! A study published by Scientific American indicates that changes to your diet can improve your gut bacteria within three or four days and it's possible to reset your hunger hormones in just three days.
I'll dive into hunger hormones more in chapter five, but know for now that these chemical messengers can play a crucial role in the effectiveness of your weight loss efforts.

This 3-Day Reset does not look like a typical weight loss protocol, and I'll be totally honest: You will not lose 10 pounds in three days. This plan is designed to get you in a better place when it comes to your food choices and catalyze many more positive changes in your belly and life. Here's what my clients Jessica and Yvonne experienced:

"Usually I give up easily on plans and protocols, but this one was different! I gave myself permission to make swaps when something didn't work for me. The end result? I lost 4 pounds of bloat!" – JESSICA

"The thing I loved most about this reset was that it was so doable. I went into it focused on ease and peace, and it really was easy to follow along without the mental chatter I often find myself sorting through. I never felt hungry, I never felt deprived or like I was restricting. I felt like I was feeding myself well and felt taken care of." – YVONNE

Here are some of the benefits you can expect to see (and feel) after completing this three-day plan:

♦ A calmer and flatter belly
♦ Less mindless snacking
♦ Feeling more confident in your meal prepping abilities
♦ And yes, you might lose some pounds

You'll notice a number of foods repeated or repurposed to minimize the total number of ingredients, allowing you to stop, drop, and do this any day of the week. For this reason I purposely kept the meals simple and flexible. I also wanted to be a responsible coach and not make this feel diet-y or cleanse-y so that you don't jump into that mind-set of "I'm starting my detox on Wednesday so until then I'll eat all the things."

Just like the Power Parfait from chapter four, this is a template for you to follow, and eventually make your own.

Heads up—the first few days of any new routine can be the most challenging. Why? Because we live on autopilot and are used to eating what's easy and what's available (or what your partner/coworker/roommate is eating). You'll need to be a little bit more proactive and thoughtful when it comes to what you're putting in your body until this new way of eating becomes second nature.

If you're not ready to do this right now, that's okay! Feel free to scan it and come back at a time in your life that feels good to you. But if you know this is what you need, grab your grocery list and commit to it now.

SET YOUR INTENTION

My favourite part of a yoga class isn't laying down at the end of class in Savasana pose (although that's great, too) but when I'm asked by the teacher to set an intention for the class. I find this moment to pause so powerful – it immediately brings me into myself and is a sweet reminder of what any act of self-improvement is about. Yoga, as well as this reset, is not just about the physical benefits; it's about taking care of yourself at a deep level.

It's also helpful to have an intention to check back in with during more challenging moments. I recommend writing down your intention then reading it daily throughout your reset. If you're following along in your workbook, use the space provided there to clearly define your intentions.

Intention: *the thing that you plan to do or achieve: an aim or purpose*

Intentions don't have to be complicated or 'woo-woo'. They simply define the way you want to feel or what you want to focus on. I encourage you to focus on a feeling rather than on a specific physical goal. Here are some examples from people who have gone through this reset:

♦ My intention is to feel more confident in my daily food choices.

♦ I want to feel like I'm taking care of myself, instead of just reaching for what's available.

♦ I hope to feel more connected to my body and my intuition.

How many times have you sworn off sugar, bread or coffee on a Sunday night and by Tuesday morning found yourself grabbing a granola bar with a giant latte as you rush to the office?

Take a step back and ask yourself: how do I want to feel? What is the root of my desire to eat healthily? Brainstorm a few feelings that you are looking to introduce into your life. And then each time you have a choice to make (Side salad or fries? Happy hour or yoga? Another coffee or herbal tea?), make the one that aligns with that desired feeling.

Freewrite for a few minutes to get all of your feeling- or word-focussed intentions out. You don't need to sum them up in a single or few words to start; just write everything down that comes to mind. After you've completed that part, go back and circle any words or feelings that jump out at you. Something that makes your heart sing or your belly feel calm would be great: intention words or feelings, for example.

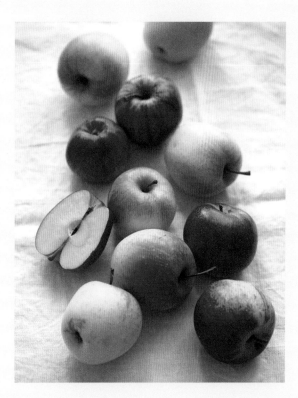

LET'S GO SHOPPING

Now that you've set your intention, it's time to get shopping! This list will be enough for one person for three days, plus some extra.

THE RESET: FRESH GROCERIES

- 1 large (32-ounce) container unsweetened plain yogurt of choice (goat's, sheep's, organic cow's, or plain coconut)
- 1 jar raw fermented sauerkraut
- Bone broth (at least 1 quart)
- 6 eggs
- Smoked salmon
- Rotisserie chicken
- 1 head green-leaf lettuce
- 1 pound carrots
- 1 avocado
- 1 bunch collard greens
- 2 bunches other leafy greens of choice (for soup—spinach, watercress, kale, mustard greens, and/or more collards)
- Medium to large piece of fresh ginger

- 1 head garlic
- 1 yellow onion
- 1 bunch scallions
- Raw Power Veggies of choice: fennel, jicama, celery, and radishes (you can get one of each, or several of one)
- 1 head cauliflower
- 1 package stir-fry veggies (fresh or frozen)
- 2 or 3 small containers fresh berries (or 2 or 3 small apples)
- 2 or 3 lemons
- 2 bottles of kombucha (or homemade Fermented Fruit Soda, page 181)
- Unfiltered quality apple juice (aim for fresh and unpasteurized)
- Organic miso paste

THE BIG KOMBUCHA QUESTION

A lot of my clients ask me about the sugar in kombucha. Is it okay? The short answer is this: It depends. For 95 percent of my clients, kombucha is key in supporting their health and helping them reduce their consumption of beverages like soda, coffee, and alcohol. But yes, sometimes the sugar is too much for certain people. It all depends on your constitution and condition.

Most of the sugar in kombucha is what feeds the living, healthy bacteria. It gets broken down and the sugar is literally consumed by the culture. However, there's always a little residual sugar.

Read your labels and pick the brands with the least amount of sugar on the nutrition facts and drink no more than 4 to 6 ounces at a time.

The only way to know if kombucha and other fermented drinks work for you is to experiment. Try drinking a small glass every day for five days and notice how it makes you feel. If you feel energized, clear-headed, and have no funny digestive stuff going on, stick with it! On the other hand, if you feel bloated, gassy, or just plain tired when you drink kombucha regularly, it may not be right for you right now.

THE RESET: PANTRY STAPLES

You may already have these on hand—
check before you start your
3-Day Good Gut Reset

- ◆ Protein powder of choice
- ◆ Chia seeds
- ◆ Psyllium husk
- ◆ Canned wild salmon or sardines
- ◆ Nori seaweed sheets
- ◆ Plain, old-fashioned rolled oats
- ◆ Sea salt and black pepper
- ◆ Za'atar spice (or curry powder)

- ◆ Cayenne pepper
- ◆ Dijon mustard
- ◆ Tamari or coconut aminos
- ◆ Coconut oil or ghee
- ◆ Pumpkin seed oil (optional)
- ◆ Toasted sesame oil (optional)
- ◆ Teas (my favorite reset teas include nettle, dandelion, and ginger)

GET YOUR RESET PREP ON

The next step is to do a little meal prep so you're not cooking everything from scratch. Here's what I suggest doing the day before you start the Reset:

1 Make your Reset Power Parfaits

For your breakfast, grab three mason jars, medium glasses, or silicone containers. Into each container put ¾ cup yogurt, ¼ cup oats, 1 teaspoon chia seeds, a small scoop of protein powder, and a splash of nut milk or water. Mix this all together and top with 1 cup berries (or chopped apple) and a generous sprinkle of cinnamon. Put lids on your containers and pop them in the fridge.

ALTERNATIVE MAKE-AHEAD BREAKFASTS

Not everyone can digest the proteins in dairy. If you can't tolerate dairy, here are a few amazing breakfast alternatives that still fit the reset plan. Just make sure to update your shopping list accordingly.

- ◆ Blueberry Pie Smoothie (page 90)
- ◆ Baked Oatmeal (page 77)
- ◆ Breakfast Salad (page 93)
- ◆ 2 hard-boiled eggs, ½ avocado, sauerkraut, drizzle of extra-virgin olive oil (bonus points if you can get some made-to-order steamed leafy greens on your plate, too!)

2 Roast your veggies

Preheat the oven to 425°F. Wash the carrots and cauliflower. Cut the carrots into sticks and the cauliflower into bite-size florets (time-saving hack: buy pre-chopped veggies). Place the carrots on one baking sheet and the cauliflower on another. Toss both trays of veggies with coconut oil and any desired seasonings. Place the baking sheets in the preheated oven and cook until the carrots are tender and the cauliflower is browned. Set your cooked veggies aside (to fully assemble your meals in advance), or store in a sealed container in the fridge.

tip

Line your baking sheets with parchment paper or aluminum foil for easy cleanup!

3 Wash and prep your greens

Wash your greens well (all of 'em!) and then pat dry. You can also chop any leaf lettuce or kale at this point.

4 Make your Good Gut Gellies

This is the easiest prep step of all: in a medium container, combine 1½ cups apple juice and 6 tablespoons psyllium husks. Mix well and divide evenly among three small containers. Place in the fridge to firm up. Note: If you forget this step, no problem—you can make the Gellies and let them set for a few minutes and they'll still be good to go.

5 Make my Healing Greens Soup

This soup comes together in just about 20 minutes, but if you're like me and want dinner done in five, you'll want to make this in advance. You can find the recipe on page 112.

Extra credit
You can also prep your lunches in advance by filling three large to-go containers with the ingredients for each meal listed in the plan that follows.

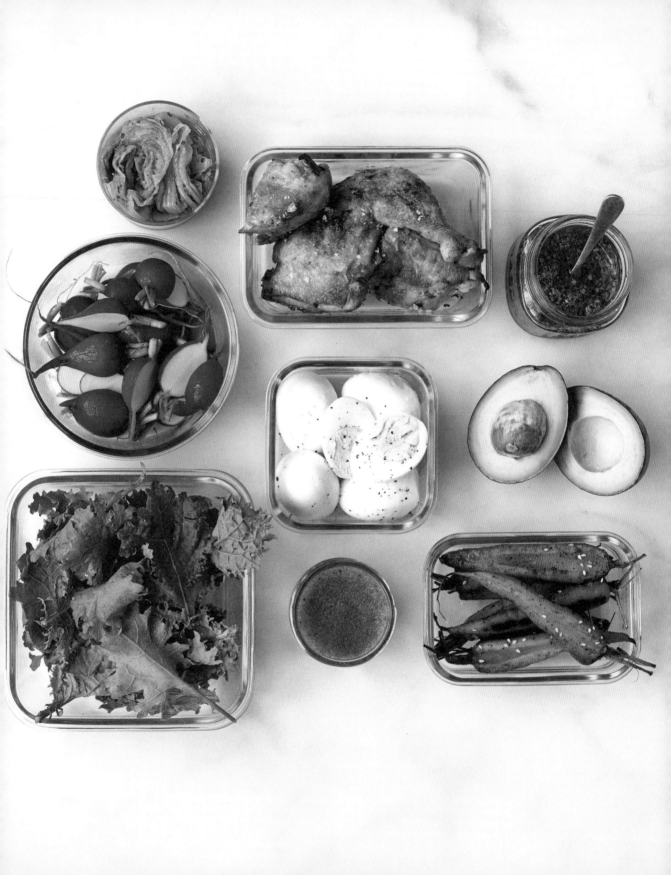

THE 3-DAY MEAL PLAN

DAY 1

AM: 4 to 6 ounces hot water with lemon and 24 to 32 ounces regular water with a pinch of sea salt

Breakfast: Reset Variation of Power Parfait (see page 44), tea or coffee with 1 teaspoon coconut oil or ghee mixed in

Optional Probiotic Pick Me Up: 4 to 6 ounces Kombucha or Fermented Fruit Soda (page 181)

Lunch: A Good Gut Rule of Five plate (see page 26) Plate: Green-leaf lettuce (as much as you'd like), about 1 cup roasted carrots, small can of wild salmon or sardines, ¼ avocado, and sauerkraut. Dress up your plate with juice from the sauerkraut, a light drizzle of olive oil, and a squeeze of lemon juice, and season with salt and pepper. I also like to add a dollop of Dijon mustard for salmon and roasted veggie dipping fun.

Snack: 1 cup bone broth and about 1 cup roasted cauliflower

Dinner: Healing Greens Soup (page 112) with an egg (cooked however you'd like) and a drizzle of toasted sesame oil

After-Dinner Treat: Good Gut Gellie (page 44) and herbal tea

DAY 2

AM: 4 to 6 ounces hot water with lemon and 24 to 32 ounces regular water with a pinch of sea salt

Breakfast: Reset Variation of Power Parfait (page 44), tea or coffee with 1 teaspoon coconut oil or ghee mixed in

Optional Probiotic Pick Me Up: 4 to 6 ounces Kombucha or Fermented Fruit Soda (page 181)

Lunch: Collard Salad Wraps with smoked salmon or turkey and avocado (page 100)

Snack: Mug of Healing Greens Soup (page 112), sliced Raw Power Veggies (as much as you'd like)

Dinner: A Good Gut Rule of Five Plate: Pile of steamed greens (as much as you'd like), ¾ to 1 cup shredded rotisserie chicken (or two hard-boiled eggs), about 1 cup roasted carrots, sauerkraut, drizzle of pumpkin seed oil

After-Dinner Treat: Good Gut Gellie (page 44) and herbal tea

tip
Have fun with your bone broth! I love adding torn nori sheets, a scrambled egg, or a spoonful of coconut oil or ghee.

DAY 3

AM: 4 to 6 ounces hot water with lemon and 24 to 32 ounces regular water with a pinch of sea salt

Breakfast: Reset Variation of Power Parfait (page 44), tea or coffee with 1 teaspoon coconut oil or ghee mixed in

Optional Probiotic Pick Me Up: 4 to 6 ounces Kombucha or Fermented Fruit Soda (page 181)

Lunch: Green-leaf lettuce or baby spinach (as much as you'd like), ¾ to 1 cup rotisserie chicken (or tinned sardines), about 1 cup roasted cauliflower, sauerkraut, squeeze of lemon juice, drizzle of extra-virgin olive oil, sprinkle of cumin, salt and pepper

Snack: ½ avocado and Raw Power Veggies (as much as you'd like)

Dinner: Bowl of bone broth with 1 cup or more of stir-fry veggies and an egg cooked in, drizzle of tamari or coconut aminos, sesame or coconut oil, and cayenne (optional)

After Dinner Treat: Good Gut Gellie (page 44) and herbal tea

RESET REFLECTION

Now that you've completed your reset, let's take a few minutes to reflect on your experience:

♦ How did this go for you? Was anything challenging? Were some times of day or meals easier than others?

♦ Is there anything you want to bring into your regular everyday routine?

♦ Would you do this again? Would you change anything? (Ask your intuition this question!)

♦ How does your belly feel? Any changes in your digestion? Energy? Mood?

Share a positive thing you learned or felt in the *Thin From Within* Book Club Facebook group!

My hope is that you will be feeling better after just three days, whether it be energetically, emotionally (that you did something for you!), or physically. For many of my clients, I suggest doing this gentle three-day protocol once a season, or even once a month. I recommend taking out your calendar and scheduling the next couple of times that you plan to hit reset again. Maybe even invite a friend to do it with you!

tip

Not feeling totally "reset" at the end of your three days? Feel free to keep going for an additional one to three days of gentle cleansing and see if you notice a difference then. You might also need a more customized plan for you—head to robynyoukilis.com/books for info on working with me one on one.

HUNGRY FOR MORE?

I hope this reset gave you a taste for how healthy eating doesn't have to suck—and how it can actually be delicious and super satisfying. No matter how this reset went (or didn't), I imagine you are hungry for more, ready to take the next step toward your healthiest you.

In the next chapter, I'm going to walk you through how to set yourself up for success in the kitchen every week, including my best meal prep tips, gut-healing pantry staples, and superfoods. It's what you do most of the time that will have the biggest impact on your belly and your body.

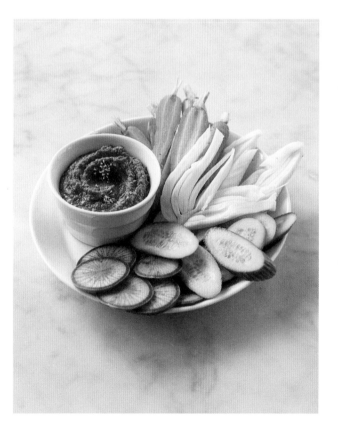

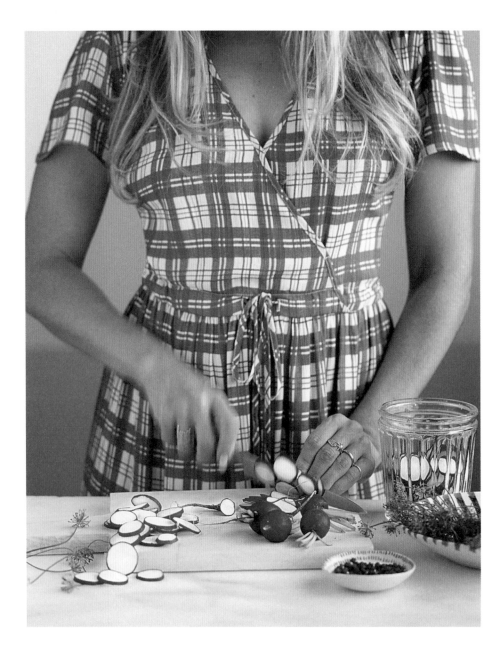

chapter five

LET'S GET
COOKING

Here's the deal: Home cooking is essential to weight loss. Cooking was the catalyst for so many changes in my body and life, and I'm confident that it can be for you, too!

Why is cooking for yourself such a big deal?

When you cook at home, you control the portions and proportions of foods on your plate and are able to load up on more of the nutrient-rich stuff (greens! healthy fats! quality protein!) your body wants and needs. Even the best restaurants typically do not serve enough veggies. I'm that girl who orders a $9 side of kale because I know greens need to make up the majority of my plate, but it's taken me some time to get to this place and it's not always easy to be the exception. Most people simply eat what's served to them, whether it's how they would build their plate at home or not.

In addition, when you make your own meals, you naturally simplify your foods and, by doing this, can more clearly hear the messages your gut is sending you about those foods. How can you expect to know what foods make you feel your best when you're not totally sure what's in your dinner because someone else made it for you? It's hard! Cooking for yourself lets you take back control and feel empowered.

Finally, when you cook at home, you naturally end up eating more high-quality food without even thinking about it. When you're constantly eating out and grabbing food on the go, you're exposed to low-quality oils, processed starches, and industrial farm-raised meat and fish. These foods can make you gain weight because your body doesn't break them down as efficiently as it does real, whole food.

HOW FAKE FOOD MESSES WITH YOUR GUT

Highly processed ingredients disrupt the natural balance of your gut bacteria and can make you bloated and sluggish. Many processed ingredients (including preservatives, fillers, and chemicals) increase inflammation in your digestive system and damage your healthy gut bacteria. In one study, a college student ate strictly fast food (filled with those fake ingredients!) for ten days. The result: His gut bacteria was devastated—about 40 percent of the species were lost.

Additionally, processed ingredients interfere with your leptin and ghrelin levels, aka your hunger hormones. I know that hormones can feel like our enemies, but you need to know about two important hormones and how they affect your metabolism and weight loss goals. Your fat cells use leptin to tell the brain how much body fat they carry. Lots of leptin tells the brain that we have plenty of fat stored (and you don't need to eat), while low levels of leptin tell the brain that fat stores are low and that we are at risk of starvation (and that you should eat). Ghrelin is a hormone made in the stomach that increases your appetite, particularly when you feel stressed. The production of ghrelin is supposed to drive us to eat, so we have the energy to handle whatever stressor is facing us.

When your leptin and ghrelin levels are thrown off, it's more difficult to know when you're hungry or full, and furthermore, if you're tired, thirsty, sad, or happy. An imbalance in these hormones also causes inflammation and digestive issues.

The good news is, when you cook more of your food at home, you're exposed to way less of the fake stuff that messes with your body's natural state of health. Getting rid of what's getting in your body's way is a big step toward feeling your best.

Small shifts in how you approach cooking can make a huge difference in how you feel—a little time in the kitchen can have a big impact on your life. Even if you usually end with #PinterestFail dishes, anyone can do a little cooking. My stories, and so many of my clients' stories, are a testament to this:

"I came home tonight and felt inspired to cook up some chicken meatballs and zoodles (also new for me) and have a sit-down dinner—party of one. I decorated the space with a fresh flower and rose quartz to make it feel special!" — GRETA

"This girl cleaned out her fridge and has started cooking with ease. I was really making everything way too hard—trapped in a spiral of my own resistance? Not every meal was perfect, but I'm annoyingly proud that I made eggs over-easy on the first try!" — MARGARET

I want cooking to feel stress-free and fun for you. In this chapter I'll help you clean out your kitchen and pantry, then walk you through what to have on hand so that cooking this way becomes so much easier.

SET YOURSELF UP FOR SUCCESS IN THE KITCHEN

Have you ever searched through your closet for what felt like forever knowing you have so many clothes but nothing to wear? Consider for a moment that your kitchen and pantry might be set up this way, too—lots of old boxes of crackers, jars of who knows what, and other mystery items that don't a meal make. When your kitchen and pantry are stocked with healthy options, you won't constantly have to weed through all the fluff to find the one thing that "fits"—all the good stuff will be at your fingertips.

THE BIG CLEAN OUT

It's time to go Marie Kondo on your kitchen à la *The Life-Changing Magic of Tidying Up* and keep around only the foods that light you up. Take everything out of your fridge, pantry, and shelves. You can do this one area at a time if that's helpful, or go all out if you're feeling fired up.

You can't have mini gluten-free brownies and veggie straws in your face every day when you want to lose weight. No, these foods aren't off limits in the big scheme of life, but for now, they need to go. Likely they're not the most supportive foods to have around on your journey.

Toss or donate anything with the following ingredients:

- Sodium nitrite
- Hydrogenated or partially hydrogenated oils
- Refined palm oil
- Cottonseed oil
- Canola oil, soybean oil, vegetable oil
- BHA or BHT
- Margarine
- Hydrolyzed vegetable protein
- Parabens
- Artificial colors and/or flavors
- High-fructose corn syrup
- Caramel coloring
- Food dyes
- Sodium benzoate
- Aspartame
- Carrageenan
- Trans fats
- Splenda
- Equal
- Saccharin
- Monosodium glutamate (MSG)
- Any of your "hot-button foods"

These are the foods that once you start eating, you can't stop. There's no concept of a serving with these foods (what, the whole bag isn't a serving?) and they often trigger other unhealthy habits. What's one of your hot buttons? Is it having peanut butter around? Do you eat the whole darn jar in one sitting? Or maybe it's bagged popcorn, granola, or raw cashews. Do yourself a favor and keep these foods out of your home, at least for now. My guess is that you'll feel lighter by simply not having these options within reach.

Toss packaged, processed foods and anything with a long list of fake ingredients. These foods damage your microbiome and mess with your hunger hormones.

You can use this clean-out time to reflect on what's going on beneath the surface that's keeping you from your goal weight. You probably know the biggest habit that needs to go before you can lose those extra pounds. If it was just about eating more piles of steamed greens and drinking water, no one would have an issue with gut health or stubborn belly weight.

WHAT ABOUT FLOUR AND SUGAR?

I'm not specifically asking you to toss white flour or white sugar, because I'm less concerned with you having these "ingredients" on your shelves than having those ready-to-eat foods that are hard to stop eating. If you want to make your aunt Susan's famous buttermilk biscuits once or twice a year with that white flour and white sugar, go for it. I'd prefer you focus on clearing out those ready-to-eat foods that don't support your gut or your mind in making the best choices on a most-of-the-time basis.

SHARE PANTRY REAL ESTATE?

If you share a kitchen, this clean-out may be a little trickier. I recommend having a conversation with your husband/partner/roommate before you toss his or her beloved cheesy poufs. Explain to them why you are doing this and keep the focus on you. Maybe you can agree to keep the foods you don't want to be eating on a certain shelf or in a basket. In fact, a study done by Cornell University research shows that you will eat the foods you can see—so if there are foods you want to avoid and you can't throw them away, hide them on the back shelf and give your roommate the map.

STOCK YOUR KITCHEN

Once you've cleared out the junk, the following list is a great place to start when you're building a healthy kitchen. You can always adjust staples to your taste, but if you're new to the healthy cooking and eating game, use this list to help take some of the guesswork out.

This isn't a weekly shopping list but rather a helpful guide to give you an idea of the produce, frozen items, and pantry staples I have on hand most of the time. The list below is organized by where I store these must-have items. For example, you don't necessarily find sourdough bread in the refrigerator section, but this is where I keep mine for optimal freshness.

tip
Choose organic versions of these staples whenever possible, and always go for GMO-free.

STOCKING YOUR EVERYDAY KITCHEN

Fridge

- Light leafy greens (like arugula, red leaf lettuce, or baby spinach)
- Dark leafy greens (like kale, Swiss chard, or collards)
- Spiralized or "riced" vegetables
- Root vegetables (carrots, beets, parsnips, sweet potatoes, and others)
- Raw Power Veggies (celery, jicama, radishes, and fennel)
- Eggs
- Tempeh
- Grass-fed butter and ghee
- Sauerkraut and fermented vegetables (raw and unpasteurized)
- Kombucha, kefir, or kvass
- Coconut water
- Apple juice or cider (no added sweetener)
- Local fermented breads (like sourdough or miche)
- Unsweetened non-dairy milk (almond, coconut, or flax)
- Yogurt
- Matcha powder (ceremonial grade)

Freezer

- Wild fish (like salmon, trout, or cod)
- Veggie burgers
- Veggies of all kinds, including "riced" vegetables
- Berries
- Cooked grains
- Portions of homemade soups and sauces, frozen in containers
- Gluten-free, sprouted breads (purchased from the fridge or freezer section)
- Dark chocolate
- Favorite raw nuts and seeds (see Tip)

Pantry

- Tinned small fish and seafood (wild sardines, wild salmon, smoked oysters)
- Jarred tuna or mackerel
- Canned or dried beans (chickpeas, black, cannellini, and lentils)
- Bean, quinoa, or brown rice pasta
- Jarred tomato sauce without sugar
- Rolled oats
- Dry grains (quinoa, millet, and amaranth)
- Onions, shallots, and garlic
- Vegetable or chicken stock
- Nut and seed butters (almond butter, peanut butter, tahini, and coconut butter)
- Gluten-free, low-sugar granola
- Simple-ingredient energy bars
- Selection of teas
- Quality sea salt and black pepper
- Favorite spices and dried herbs
- Nutritional yeast
- Apple cider vinegar
- Gluten-free soy sauce, tamari, or coconut aminos
- Oils (olive oil, coconut oil, and avocado oil)
- A variety of seaweed (nori, dulse, and snacks)
- Chia seeds
- Dried fruit (figs, dates, and goji berries)
- Collagen peptides
- Psyllium husk
- Aloe vera juice

tip

Nuts and seeds are susceptible to mold and toxins. Storing them in the fridge or freezer keeps them fresh, which means they'll be less likely to cause belly issues. For this reason, I like buying these items in small quantities from the bulk bins in busy stores.

MY FAVORITE GUT RESET FOODS

	GUT-HEALING PROPERTIES	WEIGHT-LOSS PROPERTIES	RECIPES/ USES
RAW, FERMENTED SAUERKRAUT	One of the best natural sources of probiotics. Adding 1 to 3 tablespoons to your plate at every meal will help rebalance your microbiome.	Eating fermented foods like sauerkraut can help curb cravings, especially sugar cravings, making it easier to stick to your weight loss goals.	See page 56 for more on kraut, including my favorite ways to eat it!
BONE BROTH	Full of collagen and gelatin, which help reduce inflammation in the gut and promote balance of the gut bacteria.	Bone broth is rich in protein and amino acids, which help you feel full and satisfied longer.	Drink a mug of broth for a nutrient-dense snack, use it as the base for any soup (like those on pages 112–117), or cook grains or veggies in it.
BITTER GREENS	Bitter greens (like dandelion, mustard, escarole, arugula, and the tops of root veggies like beets, turnips, and radishes) are naturally detoxifying and cleansing for your gut.	One of my favorite teachers, Paul Pitchford, says, "Bitter foods, sweet life." Our current diets tend to be so oversweetened that bitter is a taste our bodies are craving.	Honeymoon Greens (page 153), Healing Greens Soup (page 112), Blueberry-Arugula Salad (page 98), Smoked Trout and Lentil Salad (page 102)
YOGURT	Plain yogurt is rich in gut-healing probiotics. Not everyone can do dairy, so it's great that there are coconut- and nut-based options that provide lots of healthy bacteria your gut needs (see page 29).	Yogurt is also packed with protein. I find that when I eat a protein-rich breakfast, I'm full for longer and have fewer cravings throughout the day.	Power Parfait (page 36); use in place of sour cream in most recipes; Energizing Blueberry-Chia Muffins (page 85); Superwoman Bread (page 95)
COLLAGEN	Collagen is the most abundant protein in our bodies. It helps strengthen the gut lining and is great for skin, hair, and nail health—the "glue" that helps hold our body together.	Protein is a macronutrient that is essential for weight loss, and helps you stay full for hours after a meal. Collagen is a pure form of easily digestible protein.	You can buy a grass-fed powder and mix it into your morning beverage (like my Magical Morning Matcha, page 184), blend it into a smoothie, or use anywhere you'd use protein powder.

	GUT-HEALING PROPERTIES	WEIGHT-LOSS PROPERTIES	RECIPES/ USES
TEMPEH	Tempeh is naturally fermented and therefore a great gut-healing option, especially if you're vegetarian or simply want to take a break from meat.	Not only is tempeh rich in protein, but it also contains niacin and riboflavin, which help boost your metabolism.	I love to simply sear tempeh in coconut oil and gluten-free soy sauce. You can also try my Savory Sunflower Butter Tempeh (page 137).
ROOT VEGETABLES	Root veggies are super calming for the gut. For example, sweet potatoes have anti-inflammatory properties and beets are known to soothe indigestion.	They reduce cravings for white carbs since they're naturally starchy, and lessen sugar cravings because they're sweet.	Roast up a big tray of root veggies to have on hand for your Good Gut Rule of Five meals all week.
FERMENTED DRINKS	Fermented drinks, like fermented foods, pack a powerful punch of gut-friendly probiotics and offer a unique variety of different strains.	Many fermented drinks are naturally sweet and carbonated, making them healthier alternatives to soda or energy drinks.	Fermented Fruit Soda (page 181), Pineapple Tepache (page 183), Kombucha Cocktail (page 177)
FENNEL	Think of fennel as a highly nutritious, more digestible version of cabbage that can decrease bloating (rather than cause it). This veggie is highly recommended for those with IBS.	Snacking on fennel (like you would celery or carrots) is an easy way to add more veggies and crowd out junkier snacks. Plus, it really helps curb sugar cravings since it's so naturally sweet.	Slice up raw fennel for a yummy snack; Go with Your Gut Lemonade (page 180), Three-Seed Tea (page 185), Cleansing Fennel Salad (page 101), Kale Skillet Spanakopita (page 127), Veggie-Packed Meatballs (page 125)
GHEE	Ghee is easier to digest than butter since it's nearly lactose-free. It also contains butyric acid, which supports the health and healing of the small intestine.	Fat won't make you fat! It's necessary to include healthy fats in your diet for proper nutrient absorption and satiety.	Use ghee anywhere you'd use butter or coconut oil (which is likely half of the recipes in this book!).

MY LOVE AFFAIR WITH SAUERKRAUT

Sauerkraut is hands-down my favorite superfood. If you're going to pick one food from the previous list, sauerkraut is it. Is there anything sauerkraut can't do? It strengthens your immune system and provides essential B vitamins (especially B12). Plus, it will help you to curb sugar cravings and balance your gut bacteria. Sauerkraut is also high in antioxidants, which can help protect your body from developing chronic diseases.

But the number one reason I love sauerkraut is for its flavor. Kraut comes in all different varieties and is an easy way to add a serious flavor punch to any meal.

Fresh sauerkraut is worlds apart from what you might have tried slopped on a ballpark hot dog (which is always the canned variety). Raw, fermented kraut has a bright, almost lemony tanginess that's refreshing, but not sharp. When serving up a dish, think of sauerkraut as you would a squeeze of lemon or other acid. Sauerkraut (and kraut juice!) adds a zing that brightens up any meal.

You can start by buying naturally fermented sauerkraut at the grocery. It will be in the refrigerated section, and the only ingredients should be cabbage, salt, and herbs or spices like caraway seeds and turmeric. There may also be another vegetable or two.

Fermented foods, like sauerkraut, are an essential part of the Good Gut Rule of Five plate, so you'll want to experiment with adding these foods to your everyday meals.

I've even heard you can blend sauerkraut into smoothies, but I haven't tried that myself yet!

Buying sauerkraut is an amazing first step, and after that, you can take things to the next level—both in terms of flavor and gut health—by making your own. Check out the Ruby Kraut recipe on page 142. Or, you can find my basic recipe for sauerkraut in my first book or at robynyoukilis.com/books.

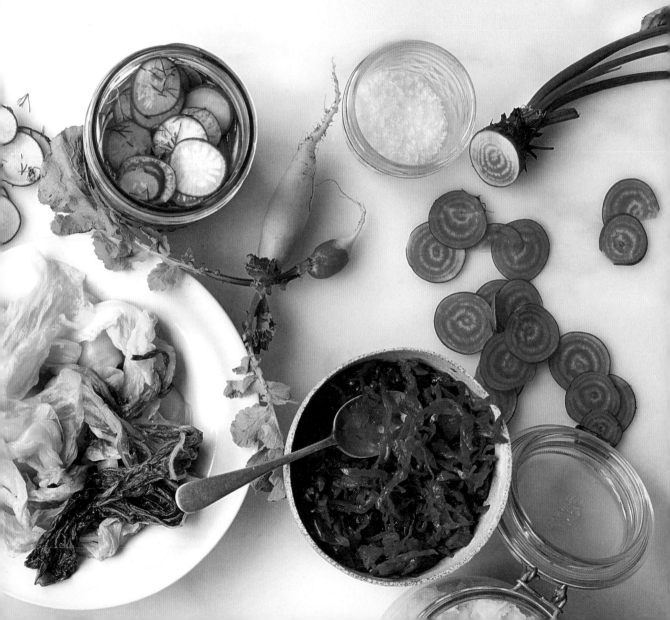

SPARKLE UP WITH SUPPLEMENTS

They say that diamonds are a girl's best friend, and I'm all about the sparkly, fun stuff, so think of supplements as the little diamonds that help your insides shine. Our nutritional needs are always changing and it's good to have some extra support.

Following are some supplement options that are supportive of your gut health and weight loss goals. I recommend trying one or two from this list and seeing how you feel. Because supplementation is such a personal topic, seek the advice of a health coach or health-care practitioner if you have any questions or hesitations before beginning any new regime.

♦ **Digestive enzymes** help you break down your food more efficiently. They add more of the natural enzymes your body produces to digest your food. Take these before meals, and especially when you're dining out or find yourself eating anything that could be troublesome for your body to digest.

♦ **Probiotics** fast-track your microbiome to be its best self. You can get probiotics from dietary sources like sauerkraut and kombucha, but it's great to take a daily dose in pill form as well (especially when following my Good Gut Reset plan). I recommend cycling your probiotic supplement to ensure you're getting a broad range of bacteria strains.

♦ **L-glutamine** is key for healing leaky gut and boosting absorption. It can repair damage to your intestinal lining by filling in the gaps that occur from undiagnosed celiac, toxins, and stress. (Head back to page 19 for more on leaky gut and other digestive disorders.)

♦ **Licorice root** (aka DGL) is my gut-healing candy! Not only is it soothing for your belly, DGL helps balance cortisol levels, which makes it especially beneficial if your gut issues have any connected emotional component (and let's be honest, whose don't?). Plus, if you like the flavor of licorice, this supplement literally tastes like candy.

♦ **Aloe vera** is a great go-to if you aren't sure what's going on with your belly but something doesn't feel quite right. It's soothing and calming. Imagine it cooling any internal sunburn (inflammation) that may be going on inside the body. Plus, it helps you poop.

♦ **Psyllium husk** is my secret weapon for my ladies who just can't go number two (or those who can go, but it doesn't feel easy or complete). Fun fact: Psyllium husk is the main ingredient in Metamucil. It's made from the husk of a plant, and it's pure soluble fiber. It promotes easy elimination by pulling waste out of the colon more quickly and efficiently. I also love psyllium husk because it's a prebiotic food.

♦ **Magnesium** is calming for your nerves, muscles, and insides. It helps with bowel movements in a really gentle way. For most people magnesium has a calming effect, but I've had a few clients who are more stimulated by it.

disclaimer
Supplements are personal to your body's needs. If you are currently taking medications, are pregnant or nursing, or have a serious medical condition, please consult with your health-care professional before starting with any new supplements.

SUPERFOODS AND ADAPTOGENS

Superfoods are nutrient-dense foods that are high in antioxidants, polyphenols, vitamins, and minerals. Really any whole food can be classified as a superfood, but here I'm talking about the extra-special ones that specifically help with your gut health and weight loss goals. Adaptogens help your body adapt to stress. This means you'll stay in the parasympathetic state more often—key for weight loss and a good gut.

If the idea of a superfood doesn't feel fun for you, feel free to skip this section for now.

These are some of my favorite superfoods for gut health and weight loss:

♦ **Chia seeds** add bulk to your digestive tract and help with good poops. They create a gelatinous mass that passes through your intestines and cleans up old waste and toxins on its way out.

♦ **Spirulina and chlorella** calm inflammation in the body and cool off stress flare-ups. You can simply add them to your smoothies or mix with water.

♦ **Goji berries** have been used in traditional Chinese medicine since around 200 BCE for their ability to generate feelings of well-being, support gut health, help build stronger muscles, and improve cardiovascular health.

♦ **Ashwagandha** is one of the key adaptogens that helps your body respond to stress. Add ¼ teaspoon to your Magical Morning Matcha (page 184) or smoothie to help stay centered and slim. Relaxation is key to losing weight and keeping any gut flare-ups or constipation at bay. Plus ashwagandha gives you a serious concentration boost.

♦ **Maca** is another favorite adaptogen for weight loss because it gives you a boost without caffeine or sugar. It also helps balance hormones, which is important in shedding those extra pounds. Oh, and it's also great for your libido. Score!

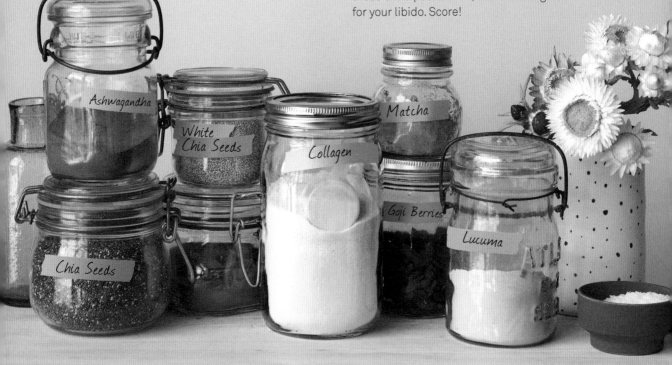

BUILD YOUR PERFECT PLATE

Your kitchen is stocked—so what's next? How do you take all these ingredients and turn them into dinner?

Sure, you can cook every meal from scratch, but I'm guessing you don't want to, or don't have time to. I'm a firm believer that a little prep planning is the first step to getting the right foods on your plate. Contrary to what many believe, meal prep doesn't have to feel like the scary, big thing that other people are capable of but you aren't. You don't have to do it all at once or lose half your weekend, and yes, it can even be fun. Armed with the right amount of meal prepping, assembling your plate according to the Good Gut Rule of Five becomes easy.

tip

A great question to ask yourself when you're considering your meal is this: How can you make it just 10 percent better? Can you use extra-virgin olive oil instead of a processed vegetable oil? Can you upgrade to organic the next time you go grocery shopping? Can you add sauerkraut? Would your tummy feel better if you left off the cheese just for today?

A quick review on what I mean by the Good Gut Rule of Five—these are the five components you want in your lunches and dinners:

1 ◆ *Greens*

3 ◆ *Protein*

4 ◆ *Fermented Food*

2 ◆ *Healthy Fat*

5 ◆ *Cooked Vegetable*

MEAL PREP FOR SUCCESS

For many of my clients, learning my easy way of meal prep is "life-changing." My client Gannon is a perfect example of what I'm talking about. "I meal prepped last night and feel so at ease knowing what I'm going to eat every day, loving what I'm eating, and confident that my fridge has enough food in it for the next week." This is what meal prep is all about—having the foods you actually want to be eating ready for you, and feeling the ease and support that comes from that.

YOUR MEAL PREP GAME PLAN

Let me walk you through exactly how to start meal prepping so you have the components of your perfect plate ready to go when you are.

Here are the basics you'll want for each week.

This list may look familiar—if you've done the Good Gut Reset (see chapter four), you've gotten a taste of what my meal prep game plan looks like. That was the point!

If you can't commit to this whole list right away, feel free to start with just one item from the list and build from there.

1 Roast a tray (or ideally two) of vegetables

I always try to make one heartier, starchier veggie, like sweet potato or winter squash, and one other cooked vegetable, such as Brussels sprouts, broccoli, or cauliflower.

Preheat the oven to 425°F. Chop your veggies of choice into equal-sized pieces, or as close as you can get. Arrange them in one layer on a baking sheet. Toss to coat with melted ghee or coconut oil, or avocado oil, and then sprinkle with salt and pepper. Roast for 25 to 45 minutes, until tender all the way through and slightly browned, flipping once. Store in glass containers (check out my favorites in my online shop at robynyoukilis.com/books).

2 Wash and prep your greens

The difference between me eating greens and not eating greens is having them washed, chopped, and ready to go. Yes, you can buy the prewashed and prechopped bags of greens, but fresh is best (for taste and nutrition). In addition, many bitter greens (included in my Favorite Gut Reset Foods for Weight Loss List on page 54) need an extra rinse to remove stubborn grit, so you're less likely to find them in your grocer's prewashed section. You might as well buy yourself a salad spinner and make this a part of your weekly routine.

Put the greens in a big ol' bowl (or salad spinner) and fill with water. Imagine that you are giving them a bath—use your hands to give them a little shimmy shake. Drain the water, rinse out any grit at the bottom of the bowl, and give the greens another dunk if needed. Spin the greens dry in a salad spinner, or lay them out on a kitchen towel and pat dry. Chop and store in reusable produce bags with a dry paper towel (to absorb excess moisture).

WHOLE GRAINS?

If your family runs on carbs (I know my husband does!), make a big batch of a whole grain (quinoa, rice, barley, farro, etc.) at the beginning of the week, too. I use my rice cooker—perfect quinoa every time! Alternatively, you can buy precooked grains in the freezer section of most grocery stores these days.

3 Prep 1 or 2 proteins of choice

I always have at least one or two easy ready-to-eat proteins in my fridge or pantry. I've included a few ideas here—some of these are recipes, and some are quicker, pre-cooked options.

Easy protein recipes:

♦ Rotisserie chicken—Either roast it yourself, or you can totally buy one from the grocery store! Just check the label for funky ingredients: It should only have olive oil, lemon, and natural herbs listed—no preservatives, margarine, or ingredients you can't pronounce. Head to robynyoukilis.com/books to download my simple whole roasted chicken recipe.

♦ Seared tempeh

♦ Hard-boiled eggs

♦ The Simplest Salmon (page 124)

♦ Grilled shrimp

♦ Veggie-Packed Meatballs (page 125)

Pre-cooked or grab-and-go options:

♦ Smoked salmon

♦ Veggie burgers

♦ Jarred tuna or mackerel

♦ Tinned fish such as sardines, smoked trout, and oysters (buy BPA-free tins)

4 Make 1 or 2 fun dressings or condiments

Dressings and condiments are what make meals fun and next-level delicious. You can use them in salads and grain bowls, or with a simple piece of fish and roasted veggies.

♦ Roasted Shallot Vinaigrette (see page 102)

♦ Beet Hummus (page 000)

♦ Amped-Up Ketchup (page 000)

5 Make a fleet (3 to 5) of Power Parfaits

Like I mentioned in chapter 3, my Power Parfait was the game-changer for me once I had my daughter, Navy, and I get messages every day on how this yummy breakfast has transformed mornings. Head over to robynyoukilis.com/books for a full step-by-step video bonus!

6 Stock your snacks and treats

Well-planned snacks can keep your blood sugar balanced and prevent a binge. Here are some suggested snacks to keep on hand:

♦ Hard-boiled eggs (make and peel them in advance, then season with salt, pepper, and Italian seasoning)

♦ Organic meat sticks (check ingredients and skip those with any from the avoid list)

♦ Clean protein bars (again, check ingredients and look for something lower in grams of sugar)

♦ ½ avocado eaten with a spoon straight out of its "container"

♦ Sliced organic, nitrate- and carrageenan-free deli meat wrapped in a nori sheet

♦ Small container of plain yogurt

♦ Organic cheese sticks

♦ Apple or celery slices with single-serving almond butter

♦ Raw fennel slices

♦ Single-serving packages of raw nuts

♦ Good Gut Gellies (page 165)

tip

I keep psyllium husk and apple juice on hand so I can always have a batch of my Good Gut Gellies (page 165) in the fridge. These Gellies are the perfect evening snack—they satisfy that sweet tooth while giving you plenty of gut-friendly fiber that will help ensure you go first thing in the morning the next day.

YOUR NEW SAVING GRACE

Let me help make meal prep happen for you.

First, get clear on when you can make time to get your booty in the kitchen. Ideally take out your calendar now and look at the rest of this week and next. Sunday afternoon and evening are the most popular times for meal prep, but if you're like me and you travel a lot on weekends, you may want to set aside time on Monday or even Tuesday, or do some of this in parts throughout the week. Think about what works best for you and your life. Grab your workbook and write down when you are going to meal prep.

Next, are there any kitchen tools you need to buy to facilitate your meal prep process? Do you have storage containers, reusable veggie bags, and to-go containers for any meals that need assembling in advance? Do you want to invest in a rice cooker?

Where and when are you getting your food? Do you need to schedule a trip to the grocery store or farmers' market? Are there any specialty items or superfoods you'll need to order online? If the thought of making a trip to the grocery store makes you tired, I suggest looking into grocery delivery services—between running my business and being a mom, it's always worth the small delivery fee for me to have my groceries brought to my doorstep.

Finally, how can you make your meal-prep time more fun? Do you need to download a podcast or audiobook, or throw on an awesome playlist? Would it help to have a cute apron to wear, or a new set of dishes?

DON'T GO NUTS

I've said it before, and I'll likely say it in every book I write: Nuts are not popcorn! Nuts are not something to eat by the handful. Notice how they come from trees in those hard-to-crack shells? That's because nature didn't intend for us to gobble them up in large quantities. Nowadays they're almost too easily available, in nut butter form, shelled and in bulk, and since they're so delicious, we tend to overeat them. They are healthy, but in reasonable portions. For this reason, I recommend buying single-serving packages of nuts or serving them in small single-serving ramekins or other small dishes.

I get that meal prep may not be glamorous, catchy, or cover-of-the-magazine cute. It's about getting in the kitchen and getting your hands and baking sheets dirty (schedule your manicure for the next day!). But the results are worth it. Think of that OMG moment when you open your fridge and it's full of foods that are ready to go when you are. It's the best feeling!

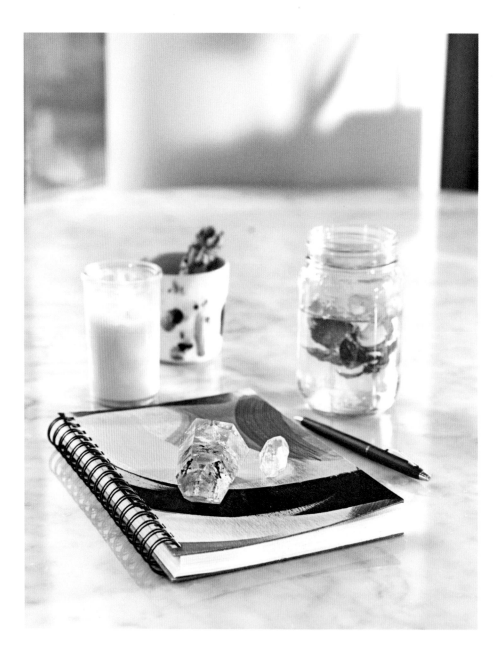

chapter six

FINDING YOUR INTUITIVE FOOD VOICE

Thus far, we've talked mostly about what to eat. How you can eat is just as important, if not more.

Your body is not designed to digest food if you're stressed or distracted. In chapter three we learned that your body has two main states: rest and digest (parasympathetic), and fight or flight (sympathetic). You are physically not able to be in both stages at once. If you are stressed out while eating (or right after you eat!), your body can't digest your food, which leads to weight gain and poor digestion.

You're better equipped to connect with your intuitive food voice and your body's natural hunger and satiety signals when you are present with your meals. When you tune in, you'll hear the signals your gut is sending you—when it's hungry and when it's full.

What if "mindful eating" just doesn't seem to happen in your day-to-day life? You have e-mails to respond to, kids to drop off and pick up, friends to call, and the list goes on. While eating mindfully can seem like a good idea in theory, it's not always easy to bring into your reality.

I get it. I knew about the benefits of mindful eating for years before my daily practice finally clicked into place. How did I do it?

In my coaching practice, Your Healthiest You, I developed my 123 Food Freedom Tool, and this three-step process to mindful eating was featured in my first book, *Go with Your Gut*. The 123 Food Freedom Tool will help you slow down at meals, enjoy your food more, and say good-bye to annoying digestive issues like bloating and heartburn.

A MINDFUL EATING PROGRAM

I'm including this tool here again because it's so foundational. It's one of the best ways to transform your eating experience without actually changing any of the foods on your plate.

My 456 Eat and Complete Practice is the next phase in my approach to shedding extra pounds that aren't you. I like to think of this as my post-meal meditation. This practice will help you drop into your parasympathetic nervous system, get clear on which foods are serving you, and address any emotional issues that may be causing you to overeat.

If you've been using the 123 Food Freedom Tool, you can add in the 456 Eat and Complete Practice right away. You can also start using both of them, and you'll notice a huge difference in how you feel in your body.

You've heard about intuition, right? This magical thing that's meant to guide us? Well, your intuitive food voice is what your gut (all those bacteria in your physical gut and your intuitive gut instinct) is telling you to eat and what to avoid.

"It's incredible what just a few days of changing your habits can do for you. Not only do I feel healthier in my body, but I feel clearer in my mind—I've been more productive at work! I'm also more in tune with my body and what it wants. I went to this health food store yesterday and browsed through the 'healthy' snacks and chocolates. Usually, I would crack and buy something but yesterday I heard a clear 'no' from my gut and I listened and I walked away. It was actually easy!" — MAUD

THE 123 FOOD FREEDOM TOOL

♦ **Step 1: Look**
When was the last time you allowed your eyes to take in the experience of eating? Eating is a complete sensory experience, and if we don't include one of our most vital senses—our sight—we are out of touch with the idea that we have eaten. Next time you're about to consume something, take a moment to take it in with your eyes. Yes, you'll want to do this with the beautiful recipes you make from this book (like the Smoked Trout and Lentil Salad on page 102), but also with simple snacks and less glamorous, on-the-go bites.

♦ **Step 2: Breathe**
Before you have your first bite, take a deep belly breath or two. Taking a good, deep breath brings you into the present and into your body again (which is necessary because you're about to use your body to eat!). Feel your belly expand and release and the gentle ahhh that comes with that simple action.

♦ **Step 3: Chew**
Chewing is so important that I created an entire free online coaching program around this practice. You can join us anytime at www.thechewingchallenge.com. The goal? To chew each mouthful completely (i.e., until it becomes liquid!) before swallowing. When you chew your food thoroughly, you stimulate your digestive juices to better process your meal. Plus, you'll naturally slow down and likely eat a little less.

THE 456 EAT AND COMPLETE PRACTICE

♦ **Step 4: Rest and Digest**
After you've used your 123 Food Freedom Tool at a meal or snack time, it's time to digest. This means spending an extra minute or two or ten (the more the better!) sitting with your empty plate or bowl after you've completed your meal, just taking that time to breathe and be.

I know that finding real time to eat may already be a stretch, so asking for an extra minute might feel completely unattainable, but I know you can do it. You can shift your mind-set from "There's no way" to "I am going to try." Plus, it takes about 20 minutes for your body to register that it's full, so you need to give your gut time to send those full signals to your brain so you aren't jumping out of your seat to help yourself to seconds and thirds that you aren't really hungry for.

♦ **Step 5: Mark the End**
You wouldn't write a sentence without punctuation and you shouldn't leave a meal without marking the end. Maybe you just take a deep belly breath to say thanks: to your food, your body for digesting, or whoever cooked—even if that's yourself.

You can also mark the end of a meal by clearing the table, putting leftovers away, and washing dishes. If someone else is on dish duty (lucky you!), make a cup of digestion-friendly tea (like my Three-Seed Tea, page 185).

♦ **Step 6: Pause and Reflect**
The last step in the 456 Eat and Complete Practice is to notice how you feel. Are you still hungry, satisfied, or overly full? What's going on in your brain? Are you judging yourself for what you just ate? Take a minute to feel out what's going on in your body and become conscious of the experience between you and your food.

FINDING YOUR INTUITIVE FOOD VOICE

We're fed so much information about diet and lifestyle trends that it's easy to get confused and stuck under the layers of opinions out there, whether it's *Vogue* magazine recommending what to eat, your best friend's latest diet, or your yoga instructor's thoughts about smoothies and juices.

You can learn the recipes, the tools, and the tricks, but this will never become part of you until you learn to listen to your own body, to connect to your own inner guru, your own intuitive voice.

This inner knowing is what takes the power away from the birthday cake, the third glass of wine, or whatever "hot-button food" you want to eat. This is your internal compass that will steer you back to you. Check in, again and again, and again.

The 123 Food Freedom Tool and 456 Eat and Complete Practice will help you slow down and connect to your own intuitive food voice. (I promise, it's in there!)

I highly recommend writing down what you notice in a journal. Not only will this strengthen your intuitive food voice, but you'll also have a paper trail to reflect on. From this you can identify any foods or situations that aren't serving your gut health and weight loss efforts.

Also, if you're sipping tea and writing in your journal, you're less likely to go hunting through the cabinets for chocolate or those cookies you just can't stop eating!

HOW TO FOOD-MOOD JOURNAL

Over the next two weeks, take stock of which foods make you feel fabulous, and which don't.

Grab your workbook (which you can download at robynyoukilis.com/books) and after each meal (or at the end of the day), jot down how you're feeling. Focusing on how you feel is an easy way to check in. Use specific "feeling words" that help you understand your body state, such as centered, focused, fulfilled, tired, annoyed, jittery, or happy.

Keep your journal close by to note when you have a strong positive or negative physical, mental, or emotional reaction to a certain food or food combination. You may feel fine right after a meal but later feel bloated and moody.

For example . . .

- ♦ Do you crash soon after your afternoon paleo blondie?
- ♦ Do steamed sweet potatoes make you feel calm and energized?
- ♦ Is your daily glass of wine (or two) totally draining your energy the next morning?
- ♦ Does gluten make your tummy feel all funny and unsettled?

Don't forget to track your "wins," too! If you have roasted squash at night with dinner and notice you're sleeping deeper, great! If you suspect that your salads are not filling enough, i.e., you still want a bag of pretzels at 2 p.m., make note of this and see if you can make a bigger portion next time and if you followed the Good Gut Rule of Five.

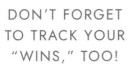

DON'T FORGET
TO TRACK YOUR
"WINS," TOO!

You can also use your Food-Mood Journal to reflect on other habits or life factors that may be helping (or hurting) your weight loss goals. Is it easier to feel satisfied by your lunch when you take it outside? Are you able to skip that second glass of wine when you take YOUR minute for you when you get home from work? Or maybe you find yourself with a stomachache every time you have dinner with a certain friend, or at the bottom of a jar of almond butter anytime after you look at your bank statement?

These are just a few examples of what you might uncover as you observe your body, but they're just that—examples. Perhaps every single one I mentioned is the exact opposite for you! The more you practice checking in, the easier it will be to identify the foods that support you best.

 Download your free Food-Mood Journal template at robynyoukilis.com/books.

A NEW BREED OF BALANCE

How many times have you heard someone say, "Just eat a balanced diet"? The big question is, how do you know when you've finally reached this heavenly realm of balance? So many of us are striving so hard to find a sense of balance in our food, and our lives, but it almost feels like we can never quite get there. Why? Because we're constantly comparing ourselves to other people. You, your BFF, your mom, and that girl you follow on social media all have different needs for a balanced diet.

For example, some of us can handle some processed foods and caffeinated drinks while others can't. Some of us do well with animal proteins, some of us don't. It's about finding your definition of balance and sticking to rituals that keep you anchored to your intuitive food voice. This is how you know when your body can handle that amazing homemade upgraded Strawberry Shortcake (page 170) and when it needs a big plate of steamed kale drizzled with pumpkin seed oil. It's about checking in with your gut instead of ignoring it and grabbing whatever everyone else is.

You may think your intuitive food voice only wants pizza and peanut butter cups (or peanut butter cups ON pizza?), but I promise it has more wisdom than that. It's time to stop comparing and despairing, and start using and trusting your gut to find your definition of balance.

BECOMING A WELLNESS BABE

What keeps us from feeling happy and at home in our bodies, regardless of the number on the scale, are the heavy thoughts of what *used to be*. A dress size. A diet. An ex-boyfriend. An old job. Holding on to that used to be mind-set will keep you feeling stuck no matter how much progress you've made.

When my client Eliza came to me, she was in a rut. She was frustrated with food in general and felt like she couldn't get back to her "old self" no matter what she tried.

"I reached out to Robyn because I wanted to learn how to take better care of my body. There are so many fad diets and confusing messages out there, it's hard to know what to believe.

After working with her I got back to basics in the best way possible. I now eat the foods that make me feel good, not what I think I 'should' eat according to someone else's plan. And guess what? It works. I do feel good. I feel lighter and happier.

I've definitely lost physical weight (maybe 5 to 10 pounds? I no longer weigh myself!), but it's so much more than that—it's the 'emotional weight' that was bogging me down. I didn't try to lose weight or count calories, but instead I focused on nourishing my gut and nurturing myself every single day."
— ELIZA

Eliza is my definition of a wellness babe. Her biggest transformation wasn't that she was able to fit in her size whatever jeans again, but that she discovered a new, even more brilliant version of herself.

Just as with Eliza, your body will naturally adjust to crave the foods that are best for you as your intuitive food voice strengthens. It will no longer be an excruciating decision-making process. More and more you'll just know.

Becoming a wellness babe is about knowing what makes you feel good now. It's about identifying your hell yes's and your no thank you's. It's about continually checking in and knowing when you can say, "I'll have what she's having" and when you affirm, "This is what I need today." It's about getting clearer and clearer on what you want in your life and soaring from that place of intuition.

And that is how you become "thin from within." It all begins with you.

Love your guts,
Robyn

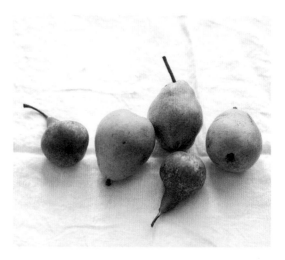

INTO THE KITCHEN

My entire journey into health and wellness started because of my deep love of food.

Any way you slice it, **food equals love.**

Whatever challenges, struggles, or confusion you've had with cooking and food, the bottom line is that food is a way we show love, and also how we receive it. I grew up in a home where this was all too true. My mom always cooked delicious meals for our family—as I've mentioned, coq au vin was a regular Wednesday night meal in our home. Her food was infused with love. I bonded with my dad over giant soft pretzels, and my brother and I had a ritual of getting Vanilla Coke floats together.

If you want to look or feel a certain way, you must get in the driver's seat of your life, and you must get in the kitchen.

We've talked about all the ways home-cooking supports your gut health and weight loss goals— when you cook for yourself you can load up on more of the good stuff and control the ratio and portions of the foods on your plate (hello, Good Gut Rule of Five!). You also naturally end up with more high-quality foods when you cook at home as well as fewer processed foods (which throw off the delicate balance of your gut bacteria and sabotage your weight loss goals). But the most important reason of all is the simple fact that there's no better way to sharpen your intuitive food voice than by getting creative in the kitchen.

Whether you're totally at home roasting trays of veggies in your oven or you currently use it to store pots and pans, I encourage you to cook the recipes in this book like the most fun, messy, and delicious challenge that you've taken on in your life.

It's time to drop the pressure of perfection and pick up the fork of pure pleasure and dive in!

Let's eat!

◇

IF YOU WANT TO LOOK
OR FEEL A CERTAIN WAY,
YOU MUST GET IN THE
DRIVER SEAT OF YOUR LIFE
AND YOU MUST GET
IN THE KITCHEN.

THE
RECIPES

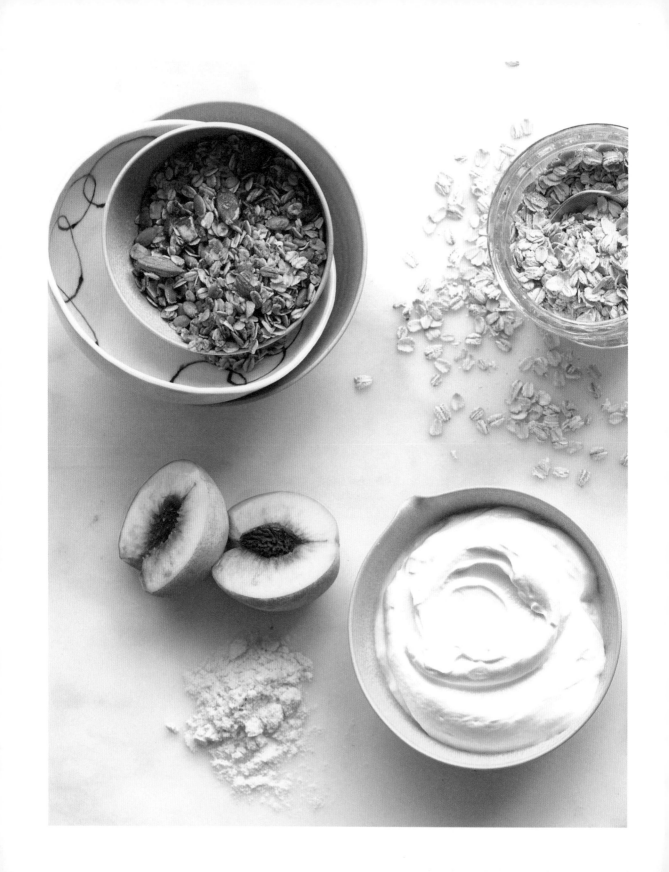

◇

MORNING
START

———

◇

PUMPKIN BREAKFAST COOKIES

This is your all-in-one breakfast to-go that you can bake, store, and eat all week. Freeze them and they'll last even longer! Just take one out of the freezer the night before to defrost and you'll wake up to a sweet breakfast that's literally ready when you are. The best part? These babies cover all your macronutrient needs—protein, fiber, and healthy fats—plus, they taste amazing. Bonus: I love them for an afternoon treat, too!

---

makes 12 large cookies

Coconut oil to grease the baking sheet
(if not using parchment paper)

½ cup almond butter

½ cup pure pumpkin puree

¼ to ½ cup raw honey or maple syrup,
depending on how sweet you like it

½ teaspoon pure vanilla extract

1 large egg

2 cups plain rolled oats

½ teaspoon baking soda

⅓ cup almond flour

2 tablespoons chia seeds

2 teaspoons ground cinnamon

⅓ cup raisins

⅓ cup chopped walnuts (optional)

⅓ cup chopped dates or figs (optional)

Preheat the oven to 350°F. Line a baking sheet with parchment paper or grease with coconut oil.

In a large bowl, mix the almond butter, pumpkin puree, honey, vanilla, and egg.

In a medium bowl, mix together the oats, baking soda, almond flour, chia seeds, and cinnamon.

Fold the oat mixture into the almond butter mixture.

Fold in the raisins, walnuts (if using), and dates or figs (if using).

Form the mixture into 12 balls and set them 1 to 2 inches apart on the prepared baking sheet. Flatten them slightly with your palm. Bake for 15 to 20 minutes, until golden brown.

Store in the fridge, loosely covered, for up to 1 week.

tip

REACH FOR NATURAL NUT BUTTER WHENEVER POSSIBLE, WITH NO ADDED SUGARS OR OILS.

◇

THE BEST BAKED OATMEAL

Is oatmeal your favorite breakfast? Then this recipe is for you. So many of my clients love a warm bowl of comforting goodness in the a.m., but don't have time to make it every day. Not only can you make this ahead of time, but this version of oatmeal has more protein so you're fueled no matter what your morning looks like. I like to use a muffin tin to make cute little single portions that are delicious room temperature or warmed up in the toaster oven.

serves 6

Oil, for greasing

2 cups plain rolled oats

1 to 2 teaspoons ground cinnamon

1 teaspoon baking powder

½ teaspoon sea salt

¼ teaspoon freshly grated nutmeg

2 tablespoons chia seeds

⅓ cup pure maple syrup or honey

2 large eggs

3 tablespoons unsalted butter or coconut
   oil, melted

1¾ cups milk of choice

ADD-INS

Apple Cinnamon: 1½ cups diced apple,
   2 teaspoons ground cinnamon

Blackberry Coconut: 1 cup blackberries,
   cut in half; ½ cup shredded, unsweetened
   coconut

Chai Spice: ½ teaspoon cinnamon,
   1 teaspoon ground ginger,
   1 teaspoon ground cardamom,
   shake or two of ground black pepper

Preheat the oven to 350°F. Grease an 8-by-8-inch baking dish, a pie plate, or 6 holes of a muffin tin.

In a large bowl, combine all the ingredients plus any add-ins and stir until everything is mixed evenly.

Bake for about 40 minutes if using a baking dish or about 25 minutes for muffins. The baked oatmeal is done when it turns golden brown and feels firm to the touch.

If you used a baking dish or pie plate, turn the baked oatmeal out onto a wire rack to cool, then transfer to a cutting board and cut it into 6 even squares or slices. If you used a muffin tin, transfer the muffins to a wire rack to cool. The baked oatmeal will keep in the fridge for 5 to 7 days.

GUT-HEALTHY OPTION

Soak the oats in ½ cup buttermilk and 2 cups water for 15 to 20 minutes before step 2, and forgo adding the milk.

tip

I LIKE USING SILICONE MUFFIN TRAYS AND BAKING DISHES BECAUSE THEY'RE NATURALLY NONSTICK.

◇

BIBIMBAP BREAKFAST BOWL

Game. Changer. If you're looking for something savory for breakfast instead of smoothies or yogurt, this grain-free bibimbap-style bowl will help switch up your sweet morning routine. Plus, this bowl is a perfect vessel for your homemade gut-friendly kimchi (page 147).

serves 1

Coconut oil, for frying

1½ cups cauliflower rice

2 cups greens, such as kale, baby kale, spinach, arugula

1 teaspoon toasted sesame oil, plus more for serving if desired

1 large egg

½ cup shredded carrots

½ cup bean sprouts

Easy Kimchi (page 147) or Pretty-in-Pink Fermented Radishes (page 144)

Sliced scallions

In a medium skillet, melt 1 tablespoon coconut oil over medium heat. Add the cauliflower rice and cook until warmed through, 3 to 5 minutes, then transfer it to your bowl.

Add the greens to the skillet and cook until wilted, 2 to 4 minutes Drizzle the greens with the toasted sesame oil and place in your bowl.

If necessary, melt a bit more coconut oil in the skillet, then crack in the egg and cook to your desired doneness.

Add the carrots and bean sprouts to your bowl. Top with the egg, and garnish with kimchi or fermented radishes, scallions, and more sesame oil, if desired.

tip

YOU CAN SWAP OUT THE CAULIFLOWER RICE FOR ANY GRAIN THAT WORKS FOR YOU (WHITE RICE, BROWN RICE, QUINOA, AND MORE)!

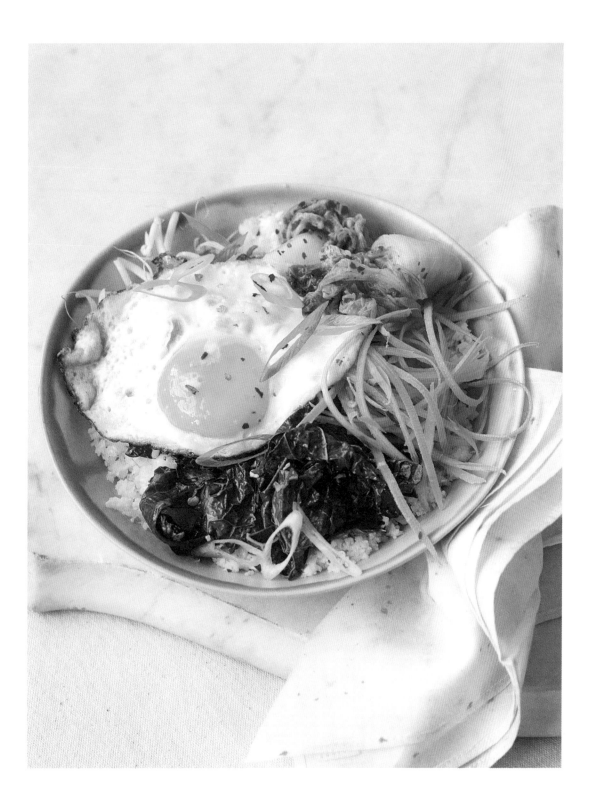

◇

HOMEMADE COCONUT YOGURT

I love yogurt and typically use goat's milk yogurt in my Power Parfait (page 36), but I know some of my community can't do dairy. This fun little mad-scientist experiment doesn't have complicated steps or require extra kitchen gadgets (except a cool thermometer!). With its good-for-your-gut probiotics and grass-fed gelatin, this yogurt is amazing for healing your gut lining, which helps you digest your food properly.

---

makes about 5 cups

3 (14-ounce) cans full-fat coconut milk

1 tablespoon grass-fed gelatin

1 to 2 tablespoons raw honey or pure maple syrup, depending on how sweet you like it

¼ teaspoon yogurt starter (available at your local health food store or online)

tip

SINCE THIS YOGURT CONTAINS GELATIN, IT DOESN'T INTEGRATE IN MOST RECIPES AS WELL AS TRADITIONAL DAIRY YOGURT. IF YOU WANT TO MAKE MY POWER PARFAIT WITH IT, I RECOMMEND BLENDING THE PROTEIN POWDER, OATS, AND CHIA SEEDS WITH THE YOGURT IN A BLENDER OR FOOD PROCESSOR. THEN SCOOP THE MIXTURE BACK INTO YOUR CONTAINER AND PLACE IT IN THE FRIDGE TO RE-SET.

In a saucepan, heat the coconut milk over medium heat until it registers 180°F on a candy thermometer.

In a small bowl, dissolve the gelatin in a small amount of water. Whisk in a few tablespoons of the hot coconut milk, then pour this mixture into the pan with the coconut milk. Remove from the heat and thoroughly mix in your sweetener of choice.

Cover and let cool to 95° to 100°F. Transfer half the yogurt mixture to a bowl and stir in the yogurt starter. Add the remaining yogurt mixture and mix well. Pour the yogurt mixture into sterilized ½- or 1-pint mason jars or other containers.

Cover and set aside to ferment at 105° to 115°F— this can be done if you put the jars in the oven and turn the light on (leave the oven itself off).

Ferment the yogurt for up to 24 hours. Taste the yogurt and see how you like it after 7 hours. When it tastes tangy enough for you, give it a stir and transfer the yogurt to the fridge. (Note that the yogurt will not thicken until it's been refrigerated for a few hours.)

Store in the fridge for up to 2 weeks.

◇

GREEN GIRL GRANOLA

If you love my Power Parfaits and want to get crafty in the kitchen making your own granola, this is my favorite go-to recipe. Cardamom is the superstar here—this Ayurvedic cooling spice has a unique taste and is great for soothing digestive issues. You can make a huge batch of this crunchy, nutrient-dense medley and store it in mason jars for weeks. Just keep it in a dry, cool area to extend the shelf life.

makes about 8 (½ cup) servings

1½ cups plain rolled oats

¼ cup flaxseeds

¼ cup hemp seeds

¼ cup pumpkin seeds

¼ cup chia seeds

1 cup dried fruit of choice (such as dates, apricots, figs, mulberries, etc.), roughly chopped

2 teaspoons ground cinnamon

1 teaspoon ground cardamom

¼ cup raw honey or pure maple syrup

2 teaspoons pure vanilla extract

3 tablespoons coconut oil or unsalted butter, melted

1 to 2 teaspoons matcha powder (optional; this gives the granola a nice green color)

Preheat the oven to 325°F.

In a large bowl, combine the oats, seeds, dried fruit, cinnamon, and cardamom and mix together.

In a small bowl, stir together the honey or maple syrup, vanilla, and coconut oil.

Add the wet mixture to the dry mixture and stir well to combine. Spread the granola in an even layer on a rimmed baking sheet and bake for 15 to 20 minutes, until golden.

Remove the granola from the oven and let cool on the pan. If using matcha, sprinkle the powder over the granola mixture and toss to combine before transferring to jars. Transfer to jars and store at room temperature in a cool, dry place for up to several weeks.

tip

HAS YOUR RAW HONEY CRYSTALLIZED? THAT'S A GOOD THING – IT MEANS YOU'VE GOT THE REAL STUFF! TO RETURN IT TO LIQUID CONSISTENCY, PLACE YOUR JAR IN A BOWL OF HOT WATER FOR A FEW MINUTES.

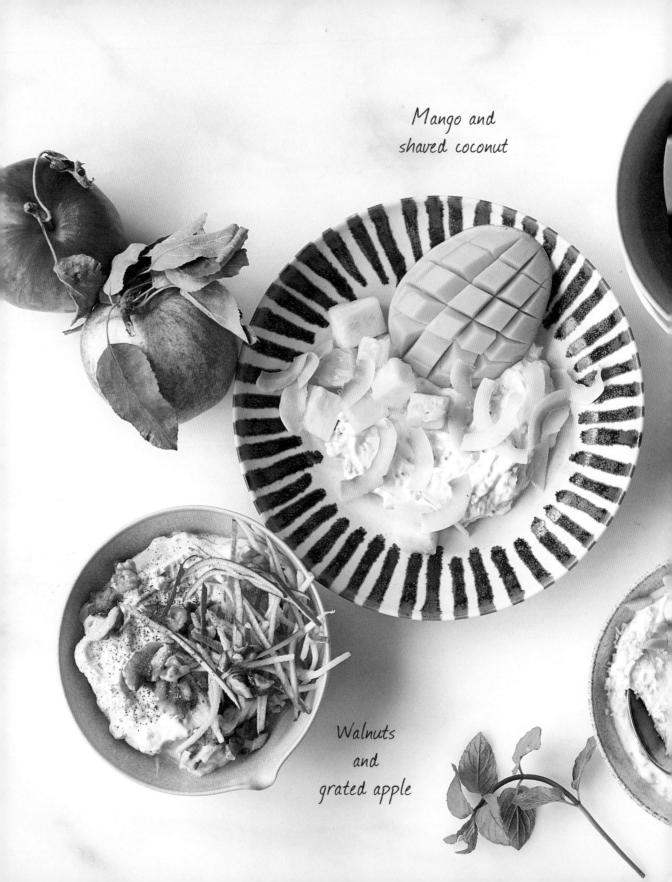

Mango and
shaved coconut

Walnuts
and
grated apple

POWER PARFAIT

FIRST, START WITH THE BASE RECIPE ON PAGE 36. THEN CUSTOMIZE TOPPINGS TO YOUR TASTE. HERE ARE SOME IDEAS TO GET YOU STARTED.

Make It Your Way!

Fresh berry mix and mint

Mashed cooked sweet potato swirl with almonds

Nectarines, fresh figs, and almond slivers

◇

GO-GO EGG MUFFIN

These savory muffins are so much more than your typical egg cup—they taste more like a muffin as opposed to a handheld frittata. Not only are they packed with veggies, but the addition of almond flour makes them feel more substantial. Pop a few of these in a storage container for a breakfast on the go. They also make for a protein-filled snack.

makes about 8 muffins

2 tablespoons coconut oil, melted,
    plus more for greasing
2 cups grated vegetables (I recommend
    zucchini, carrots, and parsnips)
2 large eggs
1 cup almond flour
¼ teaspoon baking soda
¼ teaspoon baking powder
½ teaspoon sea salt
¼ teaspoon freshly ground black pepper
1 tablespoon Italian seasoning

Preheat the oven to 350°F. Grease 8 wells of a standard muffin tin.

In a large bowl, combine the grated vegetables, eggs, coconut oil, almond flour, baking soda, baking powder, salt, pepper, and Italian seasoning. Mix until combined.

Pour the batter into the prepared wells of the muffin tin and bake for 20 to 25 minutes, until golden brown.

Store in an airtight container in the fridge for up to 4 days.

◇

BLUEBERRY
CHIA MUFFIN

I'm a Long Island girl who used to go to the strip mall for giant, white flour–laden blueberry muffins the size of my head. I still love real muffins, so I wanted to come up with a healthy version that's just as yummy without the sugar crash. Make a batch of these in advance for quick breakfasts and treats throughout the week. They also freeze beautifully.

makes 12 muffins

⅓ cup coconut oil, melted and cooled, plus more for greasing

¼ cup milk of choice

2 large eggs

1½ cups thick, Greek-style yogurt

1 teaspoon pure vanilla extract

2 cups gluten-free all-purpose flour blend

½ cup coconut sugar

2 teaspoons baking powder

Pinch of sea salt

¼ cup chia seeds

¼ teaspoon ground cinnamon

2 cups fresh blueberries

Preheat the oven to 325°F. Grease a standard muffin tin.

In a large bowl, stir together the coconut oil, milk, eggs, yogurt, and vanilla.

In a medium bowl, whisk together the flour, coconut sugar, baking powder, salt, chia seeds, and cinnamon.

Add the flour mixture to the coconut oil mixture in three additions, mixing well after each.

Fold the blueberries into the batter and then divide the batter evenly among the wells of the prepared muffin tin.

Bake for 25 to 35 minutes, until a toothpick inserted into the middle of a muffin comes out clean. Let cool in the pan on a wire rack. Store in the fridge, loosely covered, for up to 1 week.

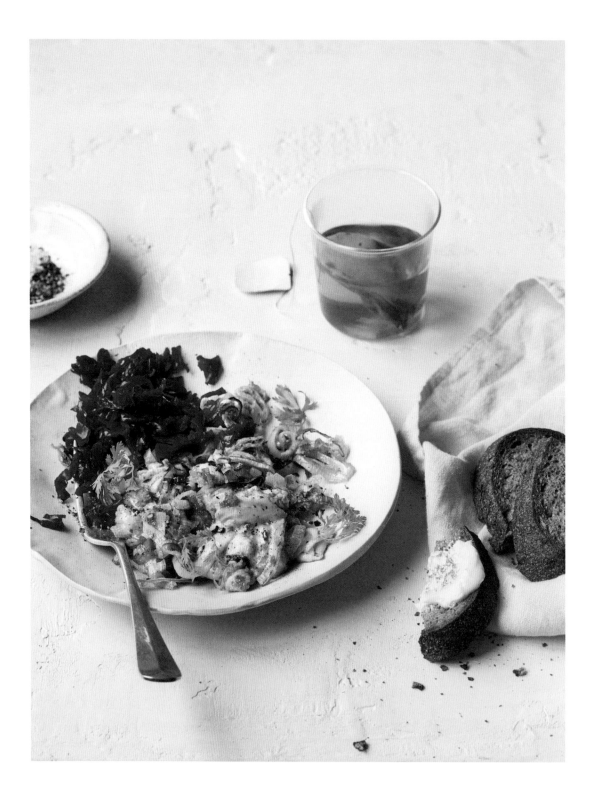

$\Diamond$

IMMUNITY SCRAMBLE

This stellar scramble recipe was developed by my cooking assistant, Gaby, and is packed with gut-nourishing, immune-boosting ingredients such as ginger, turmeric, and leeks. Fresh turmeric can turn your hands and clothes (and countertops!) a vibrant yellow color, so if you're worried about staining, I recommend wearing gloves and an apron, and using a little caution while grating the root. This delightful scramble is definitely worth the extra effort, though!

---

serves 2

1½ teaspoons coconut oil or grass-fed butter

½ cup chopped leek
  (white and light green parts)

1 (½-inch) piece fresh ginger,
  peeled and grated

1 (¼-inch) piece fresh turmeric,
  peeled and grated

4 large eggs, beaten

Sea salt and freshly ground black pepper

In a medium skillet, melt the coconut oil or butter over medium heat. Add the leek and cook, stirring, until caramelized, 5 to 6 minutes.

Add the ginger and turmeric and cook, stirring, for another minute or so, until fragrant.

Add the eggs, season with salt and pepper, and cook, stirring, until they are scrambled to your liking.

tip

FOR EXTRA-CREAMY EGGS, BRING A SMALL POT OF WATER TO A BOIL WHILE YOU'RE COOKING THE LEEKS. WHEN YOU'RE READY TO ADD THE EGGS, REMOVE THE PAN FROM THE HEAT AND SET IT OVER THE POT OF BOILING WATER—THE STEAM FROM THE WATER HEATS THE PAN AND COOKS THE EGGS LOW AND SLOW, AND THEY COME OUT SUPER FLUFFY!

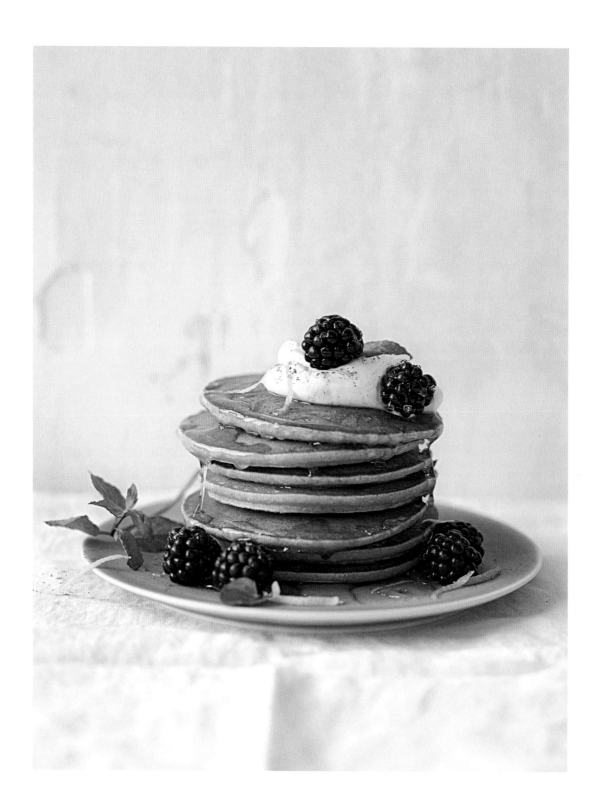

ACTIVATED CORN CAKES

Eating less gluten in our day-to-day lives doesn't mean we can't satisfy those fun, carby-food cravings—they just need an upgrade! These little guys are a great addition to your Sunday batch cooking and are so versatile. You can heat them up in the toaster oven and top with avocado, egg, and kraut for a quick lunch—just don't forget your greens on the side! Hungry at 4 p.m.? You can top one with almond butter for a perfect snack.

serves 4 to 6

1½ cups corn flour

1½ cups oat flour

1½ cups buttermilk

2 large eggs

1 tablespoon pure vanilla extract

Pinch of sea salt

½ teaspoon baking powder

¼ cup raw honey

Squeeze of fresh lemon juice

1 tablespoon coconut oil

Toppings of your choice, sweet or savory

In a medium bowl, whisk together the corn flour, oat flour, buttermilk, and ½ cup water and let sit for 10 minutes.

In a large bowl, whisk together the eggs, vanilla, salt, baking powder, honey, and lemon juice.

Add the flour mixture to the egg mixture and mix to combine.

In a large skillet, melt the coconut oil over medium-low heat. Pour ¼ cup of the batter into the skillet. Cook until bubbles appear on the surface then flip and cook on the second side until golden brown.

Go sweet and serve with your favorite pancake toppings, or experiment with everything savory.

tip

YOU CAN MAKE THE BATTER AND STORE IT IN THE FRIDGE FOR UP TO THREE DAYS TO USE FOR FRESH PANCAKES EVERY MORNING!

◇

GOLDEN MILK SMOOTHIE

This smoothie combines healing spices with lucuma, a nutrient-dense, low-glycemic sweetener made from a Peruvian fruit. Lucuma is also rich in prebiotic fiber (which feeds those good probiotics in your gut).

makes 1 smoothie

1 cup frozen steamed zucchini

1 cup nondairy milk (I recommend coconut or cashew)

1½ teaspoons chia seeds

1 teaspoon ground turmeric

1 (½-inch) piece fresh ginger, peeled

1 teaspoon pure vanilla extract

2 teaspoons ground cinnamon

1 tablespoon lucuma powder (optional)

Pinch of freshly ground black pepper

¼ cup plain rolled oats

Combine all the ingredients in a high-speed blender and blend until smooth.

◇

BLUEBERRY PIE SMOOTHIE

If banana smoothies give you a sugar high and upset your tummy, frozen steamed cauliflower is your new BFF. This secret, tasteless ingredient gives all the creaminess with none of the sugar.

makes 1 smoothie

1½ cups frozen steamed cauliflower

2 to 4 tablespoons collagen

¾ cup frozen organic blueberries

1½ cups nondairy milk (I recommend almond or flax)

½ teaspoon ground cinnamon

½ teaspoon pure vanilla extract

1 teaspoon chia seeds

1 teaspoon nut butter

Liquid stevia (optional)

Combine all the ingredients except the stevia in a high-speed blender and blend until smooth. Taste and add a drop or two of stevia, if desired, and blend to incorporate before serving.

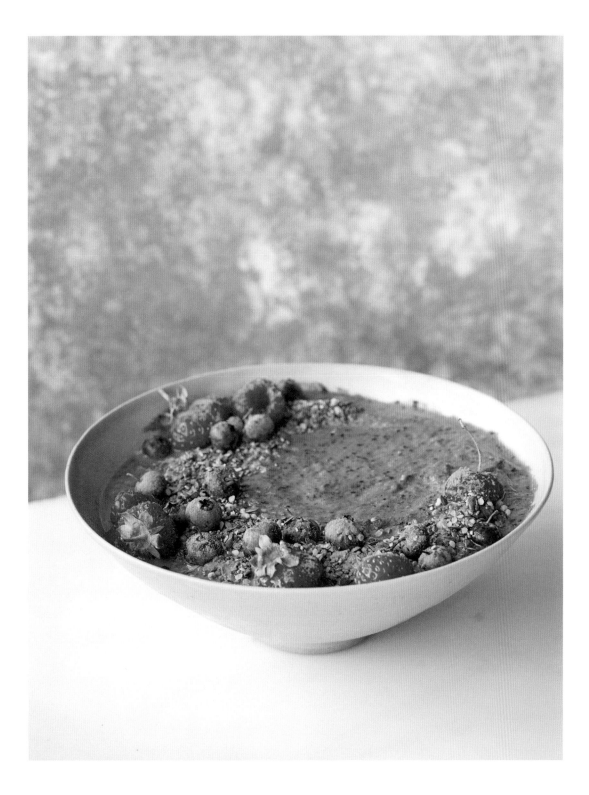

◇

NEW FAVE SMOOTHIE

This smoothie is an unusual way to use up leftover sweet potatoes, providing an easy vehicle to incorporate more of this grounding root veggie into your diet. Don't have cooked sweet potato on hand? Try subbing pumpkin!

makes 1 smoothie

½ cup cooked mashed
    sweet potato

½ large banana,
    peeled and frozen

1 cup nondairy milk
    (I recommend
    almond or coconut)

¼ cup raw walnut
    halves

Dash of ground
    cinnamon, plus more
    for garnish if desired

Small knob of fresh
    ginger (about ½ inch),
    peeled

½ teaspoon maca
    powder (optional)

1 Medjool date, pitted
    (optional)

3 ice cubes

Combine all the ingredients in a high-speed blender and blend until smooth. Garnish with an additional sprinkle of cinnamon, if desired.

◇

"PEAS, PLEASE" SMOOTHIE

This smoothie might sound a little weird, but it's actually amazingly refreshing and flavorful. Avocado makes it creamy, and peas give extra fiber. Banana sweetens it up, and all that spinach makes you feel like a green goddess.

makes 1 smoothie

¼ large or ½ small
    avocado, pitted and
    peeled

½ cup frozen peas

1 banana, peeled and
    frozen

1½ cups nondairy milk
    (I recommend almond
    or coconut)

1 or 2 scoops vanilla
    protein powder
    (2 to 4 tablespoons)

1 teaspoon pure vanilla
    extract

1 teaspoon
    tocotrienols

Generous handful
    of baby spinach

3 ice cubes

Combine all the ingredients in a high-speed blender and blend until smooth.

◇

BREAKFAST SALAD

Have you ever heard the saying, "How you do one thing is how you do everything"? Well, I like to take it up a notch and say "How you do BREAKFAST is how you do everything"! Starting your day on a healthy note has a domino effect on the rest of your day. When you start with a nutrient-dense meal, like this breakfast salad, you're way more likely to choose healthy eats all day long.

---

serves 1

Coconut oil, for frying

1 or 2 large eggs

Generous 2 cups greens, such as arugula, baby kale, or baby spinach

Good-quality extra-virgin olive oil

½ cup cubed roasted or steamed sweet potato, warm or at room temperature

Sauerkraut, for serving, plus a drizzle of the fermentation juice

¼ avocado

Gomasio (see Note), for garnish (optional)

Sea salt and freshly ground black pepper

In a small skillet, melt enough coconut oil over medium heat to coat the bottom of the pan.

Crack the egg(s) into the skillet and cook to your liking.

Put the greens in a bowl and drizzle lightly with olive oil. Toss to coat the leaves. Top with the sweet potato, sauerkraut, avocado, and egg(s). Drizzle with sauerkraut juice.

Sprinkle with gomasio, if desired, and season with salt and pepper.

tip

YOU CAN ALSO LIGHTLY STEAM THE GREENS FOR A WARMER VARIATION.

note

GOMASIO IS A JAPANESE CONDIMENT MADE OF SESAME SEEDS AND SALT. IT'S DELICIOUS HERE AS WELL AS ON SOUPS AND PLAIN COOKED PROTEINS AND GRAINS.

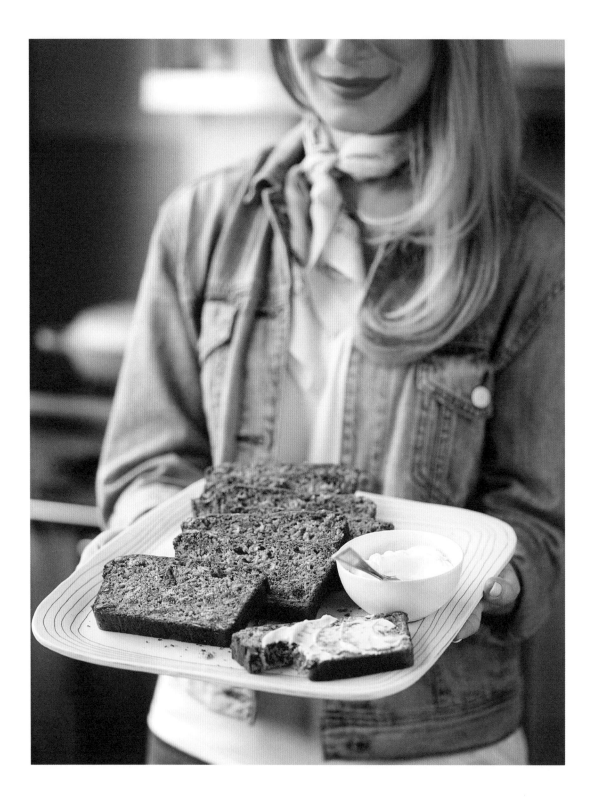

◇

SUPERWOMAN BREAD

When my sister-in-law had a baby (hi, Noa, I love you!), I made her this bread to have on hand during her marathon nursing sessions, and froze it in slices that were easy to reheat. This bread is so good for women's hormonal health, from the flaxseed meal to the goji berries. There's no kneading or complex fermentation process here, but it comes out like a real loaf of bread.

makes 1 loaf

Oil, for greasing

2 tablespoons flax meal (ground flaxseeds)

1¾ cups gluten-free all-purpose flour blend

1¼ cups rolled oats

½ teaspoon sea salt

1 teaspoon baking soda

½ teaspoon ground cinnamon

¼ cup goji berries

2 tablespoons chia seeds

2 tablespoons hemp seeds

¼ cup dried apricots, chopped

½ cup (1 stick) unsalted butter, at room temperature

3 large eggs

1 cup coconut sugar or date sugar

1¼ cups yogurt

2 tablespoons milk of choice

1 teaspoon pure vanilla extract

2 tablespoons orange zest

Preheat the oven to 350°F. Grease a standard 9-by-5-inch loaf pan.

In a large bowl, mix together the flax meal, flour, oats, salt, baking soda, cinnamon, goji berries, chia seeds, hemp seeds, and apricots.

In a separate large bowl, mix the butter, eggs, coconut sugar, yogurt, milk, vanilla, and orange zest.

Slowly add the flour mixture to the butter mixture and mix thoroughly to combine.

Pour the batter into the prepared loaf pan and bake for 1 hour, or until a toothpick inserted into the center comes out clean.

Remove from the pan and let cool. Wrap in foil or a clean dishtowel. This will keep on the counter for a day or two; you can also slice it and freeze to enjoy later.

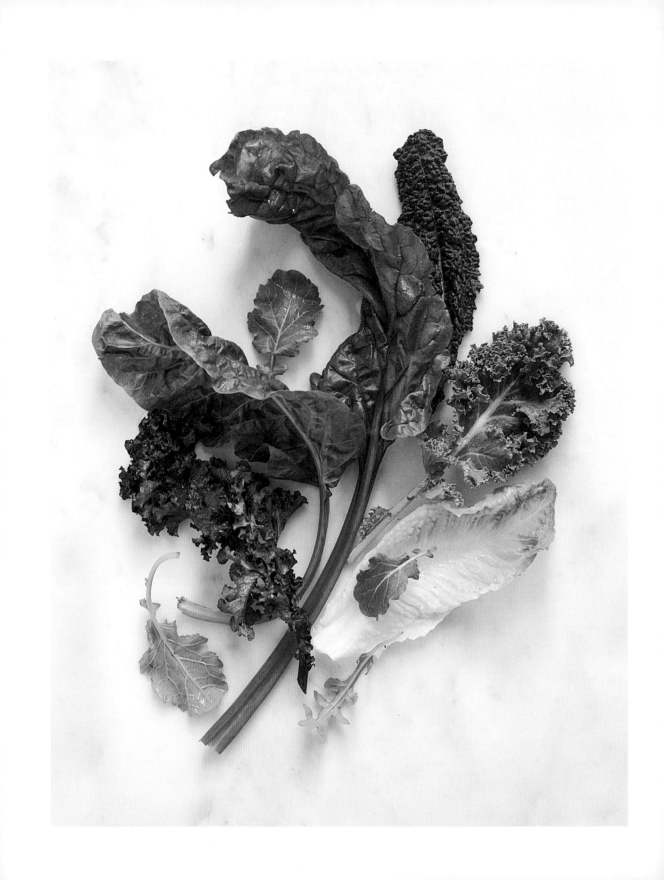

◇

SALADS
AND SOUPS

◇

BLUEBERRY-ARUGULA SALAD

My secret to the best salads ever? Add blueberries. Seriously, I could eat this salad every day of the summer and not get sick of it. It's that good! Also, I find that when I add some naturally sweet fruits and veggies to my meals, I'm much less likely to crave that "something sweet" afterward.

---

serves 1

½ to 1 cup cooked quinoa

1 (5-ounce) package arugula

2 carrots, grated or shaved

½ cup fresh blueberries

¼ cup roasted unsalted hazelnuts or
  slivered almonds

¼ cup goat cheese, crumbled (optional)

Juice of 1 lemon

2 tablespoons extra-virgin olive oil

Sea salt and freshly ground black pepper

HOMEMADE HONEY MUSTARD

½ cup plain yogurt
  (thick Greek-style works best)

3 tablespoons Dijon mustard

2 tablespoons raw honey

3 tablespoons lemon juice

¼ cup extra-virgin olive oil

Sea salt and black pepper to taste

In a large bowl, combine the quinoa, arugula, and carrots.

Top with the blueberries, nuts, and goat cheese, if desired.

For a simple dressing, toss everything with the lemon juice and olive oil and season with salt and pepper.

Alternatively, you can dress the salad with the Homemade Honey Mustard: Combine the yogurt, mustard, honey, and lemon juice in a medium bowl. Slowly add the oil, whisking constantly until well blended. Add the salt and pepper. This makes about 1 cup. You won't need all of it to dress this salad; save the rest in an airtight container in the fridge, where it will keep for up to one week.

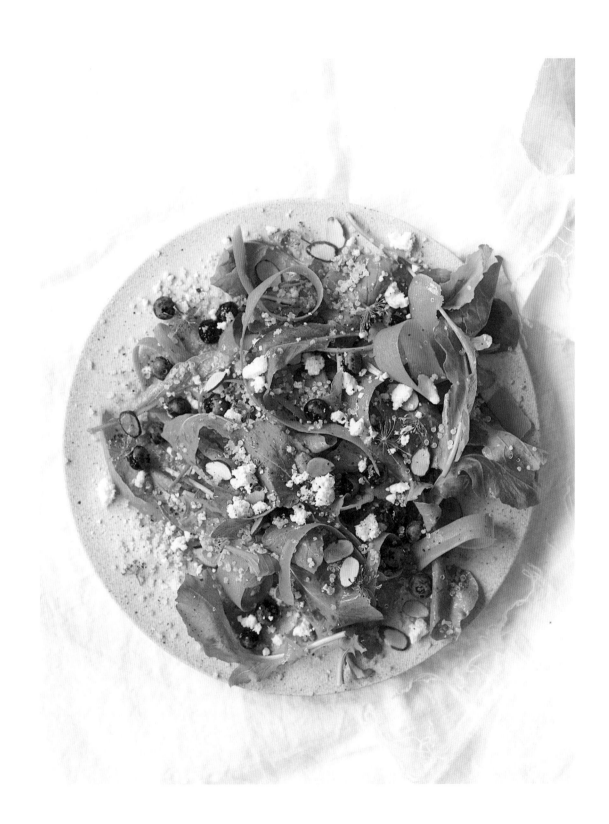

◇

COLLARD SALAD WRAPS

There's something about the combination of collard greens and naturally salty nori sheets that make these wraps oh-so craveable. These wraps meet the Good Gut Rule of Five, making them a perfect alternative to a typical salad or bowl meal. Plus, they're fun to eat! Feel free to use the recipe below as a guideline to experiment with your wrap ingredients!

serves 1

2 collard green leaves

2 to 3 sheets of nori

Optional: hummus, Beet Hummus
  (page 148), tahini, or other spread
  of choice

Smoked salmon or smoked turkey breast

½ cup roasted veggies (carrots and sweet
  potatoes are my favorites here!)

½ avocado, sliced

½ apple, cored and sliced (optional)

Sauerkraut

Fresh herbs

Wash and dry the collard green leaves and then use a knife to shave down the stem (or remove it altogether).

Lay your collard green leaves on a flat surface. Layer a nori sheet on top of each leaf. If you're using a spread like hummus, spread that over half of each wrap.

Layer on the smoked salmon or turkey, roasted veggies, avocado, apple slices, if using, sauerkraut, and herbs. You'll want to keep your toppings on just half of the wrap so you can roll it up.

Roll up your wrap like you would a burrito, folding in the bottom to keep all your toppings in. Enjoy immediately, or wrap up in foil for a quick meal on the go!

◇

CLEANSING FENNEL SALAD

Let's talk about fennel for a minute: Fennel is a celery-like vegetable with an interesting licorice flavor, and it's one of the ultimate Go with Your Gut weight loss foods. It's exceptionally high in fiber, which helps move things through your digestive tract. It's also been used for centuries after meals to prevent stomach upset. This simple salad is one of my favorite ways to highlight this underused veggie. If you eat dairy, try toping the salad with a few thin slices of Parmesan.

serves 4

1 fennel bulb, cored and thinly sliced,
   1 tablespoon fronds chopped and reserved
   for garnish if desired
2 celery stalks, thinly sliced
1 kohlrabi, peeled and cut into matchsticks
   (optional)
Juice of ½ lemon
2 tablespoons extra-virgin olive oil
Sea salt and freshly ground black pepper
Toasted pine nuts, slivered almonds,
   or pumpkin seeds, for garnish (optional)

In a large bowl, combine the sliced fennel, celery, and kohlrabi, if using.

Add the lemon juice, olive oil, and salt and pepper to taste. Toss to combine.

Garnish with the reserved fennel fronds and/or nuts before serving.

◇

SMOKED TROUT AND LENTIL SALAD

The inspiration for this salad comes from one of my favorite NYC restaurants, Café Gitane. It's the exact salad you want to eat while sitting at a sidewalk café sipping rosé. The smoked trout is full of omegas that are great for healthy skin, and the lentils will fill you up, keep you energized, and ensure your digestion is moving right along.

serves 4

SALAD

1 cup beluga lentils

½ cup cherry tomatoes, halved

½ cup crumbled goat cheese

⅓ cup walnuts, coarsely chopped

1 avocado, pitted, peeled, and diced

⅓ cup raisins or dried cranberries

4 cups arugula

2 smoked trout fillets, skins removed,
   if possible (can also swap for sardines
   or smoked mussels)

ROASTED SHALLOT VINAIGRETTE

2 medium shallots, halved

3 garlic cloves

½ cup olive oil, plus more for drizzling

Small handful of flat-leaf parsley leaves

1 teaspoon Dijon mustard

¼ cup apple cider vinegar

½ teaspoon sea salt

Pinch of freshly ground black pepper

Cook the lentils: Combine the lentils and 2 cups water in a pot over medium-high heat and bring to a boil.

Cover, reduce the heat, and simmer for 20 to 30 minutes, or until the lentils are tender. Drain any excess water.

Make the vinaigrette: Preheat the oven to 400°F. Place the garlic and shallots on a baking sheet and drizzle with olive oil. Roast until just lightly browned, about 15 minutes. Let cool slightly.

Transfer the garlic and shallots to a blender. Add the parsley, mustard, vinegar, olive oil, salt, and pepper and blend until smooth. Add a little more olive oil to thin it out, if needed.

Make the salad: In a large bowl, gently combine the lentils, tomatoes, goat cheese, walnuts, avocado, raisins, and vinaigrette to coat.

Put 1 cup of the arugula on each of four plates and top with a generous scoop of the lentil salad.

Cut the smoked trout into pieces and place on top of the lentil salad.

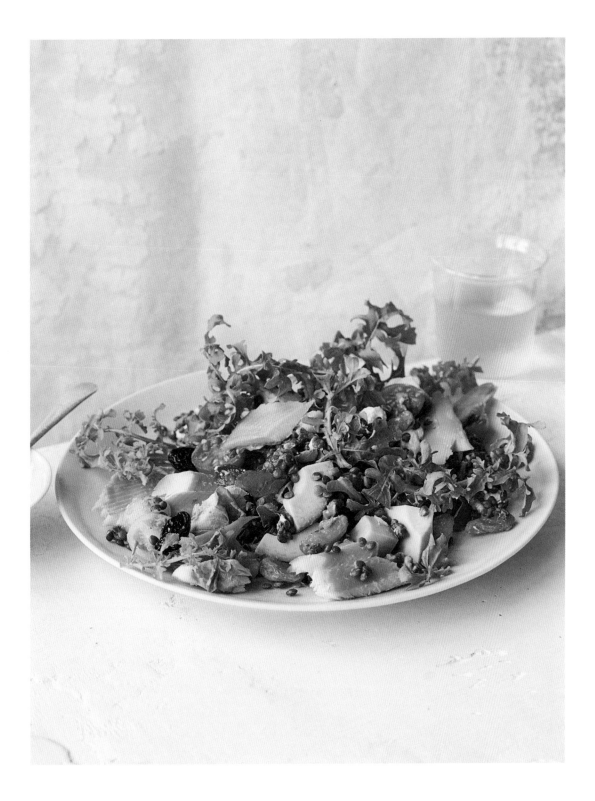

CHEEZY BROCCOLI SOUP

◇

This dairy-free soup tastes just as good (if not better) than the classic, and won't leave you feeling bloated. The secret ingredient is nutritional yeast. Nutritional yeast is a product made from deactivated yeast—it's rich in B vitamins and has a nutty, tangy flavor, which is why it's often used as a cheese substitute in vegan and paleo recipes. Bonus: Most of these ingredients are pantry staples.

---

serves 6

1 tablespoon butter or ghee

1 small onion, chopped

Sea salt and freshly ground black pepper

2 garlic cloves, minced

1 pound broccoli florets
  (from about 2 heads), chopped

½ cup nutritional yeast

Juice of ½ lemon (about 2 tablespoons)

Leaves from 1 small bunch fresh parsley,
  chopped

1 (14-ounce) can coconut milk (optional)

In a large pot, melt the butter over medium heat. Add the onion, season with salt and pepper, and cook, stirring, for 5 to 7 minutes, until softened.

Add the garlic and cook, stirring, for a few minutes more, until fragrant.

Add 4 cups water and bring to a boil. Add the broccoli and cook until bright green, 3 to 4 minutes.

Remove the pot from the heat and carefully transfer the soup to a blender or food processor (you may need to do this in batches). Add the nutritional yeast, lemon juice, and parsley. If you like the taste and creaminess of coconut milk, add that too.

Blend until smooth (be careful when blending hot liquids). Alternatively, blend the soup directly in the pot using an immersion blender.

Serve immediately, or store in an airtight container in the fridge for up to 5 days.

◇

UMAMI MUSHROOM SOUP

Mushrooms are totally trending right now. There's a reason mushrooms are so popular—they're packed with key minerals like selenium, copper, potassium, and iron. Mushrooms also are especially good if you don't eat much meat—they're rich in umami flavor, which is often missing from our diets.

---

makes 3 to 4 servings

2 tablespoons dried mushrooms (shiitake, morel, chanterelle, etc.)

4 tablespoons unsalted butter or ghee

2 leeks, white and light green parts, thinly sliced and well washed

Sea salt

4 garlic cloves, thinly sliced

5 cups fresh mushrooms (choose a combination of cremini, oyster, chanterelle, button, and/or portobello), chopped

Freshly ground black pepper

1 cup bone broth or vegetable broth

2 tablespoons chopped fresh sage

1 tablespoon fresh thyme leaves (or 1 teaspoon dried)

Splash champagne or red wine vinegar

Put the dried mushrooms in a small bowl and cover with boiling water. Let soak for 20 minutes to rehydrate. Scoop out the mushrooms and set aside. Line a fine-mesh sieve with a coffee filter and strain the soaking liquid. Set aside.

In a large pot, melt the butter over medium heat. Add the leeks and a pinch of salt and cook, stirring, for 5 minutes, or until softened. Add the garlic and cook, stirring, until fragrant.

Add the fresh mushrooms and season with salt and pepper.

Add the rehydrated dried mushrooms and their soaking water, the bone broth, and 1 cup water and bring to a boil.

Reduce the heat to maintain a simmer. Add the sage and thyme. Cover and cook for 15 to 20 minutes.

If needed, use more water or broth to thin the soup. Add a splash of vinegar. Serve the soup as is, blend it up, or blend half and mix it back in!

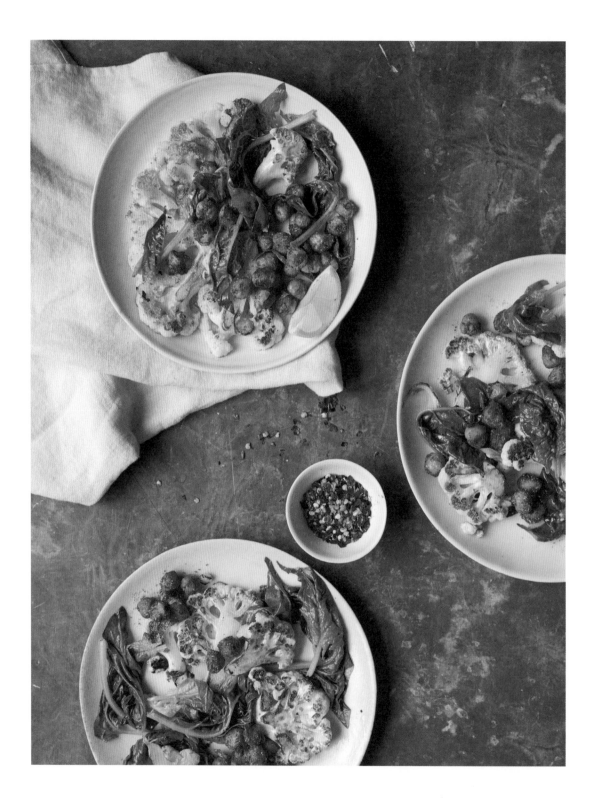

◇

WARM CAULIFLOWER SALAD

From an Ayurvedic perspective, raw foods are cold, dry, light, and rough, and consuming too much of these foods can strain our digestive fire, particularly for those who have weak digestion. This can lead to poor nutrient absorption, bloating, and discomfort. Enter: the warm salad! An easy way to make your salad more gut friendly, and especially enjoyable during colder months.

---

serves 4

SPICED CHICKPEAS

2 tablespoons olive or avocado oil

1 (15-ounce) can chickpeas, drained and rinsed

½ teaspoon ground cumin

¼ teaspoon paprika

¼ teaspoon red pepper flakes

Sea salt and freshly ground black pepper

SALAD

2 tablespoons olive or avocado oil

½ head cauliflower, sliced

1 (5-ounce) clamshell box fresh spinach

Lemon wedges, for serving

Make the spiced chickpeas: In a large skillet, heat the oil over medium heat. Add the chickpeas, cumin, paprika, red pepper flakes, and salt and black pepper to taste. Cook stirring occasionally, until crisp, 12 to 15 minutes. Transfer to a plate.

In the same pan, heat the remaining 2 tablespoons oil. Add the cauliflower and cook, stirring, until browned on both sides.

Add the spinach, return the chickpeas to the pan, and cook, stirring, until the spinach is slightly wilted.

Serve with lemon wedges for squeezing over the top.

◇

GRILLED SALAD

Grilling is an underused technique when it comes to preparing salad greens. Charring your romaine a little gives an amazing smoky, rich flavor. This is a great side dish for summer BBQs, and you can even "grill" your romaine in a skillet for a fun little dish any time of year.

---

serves 4

4 teaspoons chopped fresh herbs, such as
   rosemary, thyme, tarragon, and oregano
¼ cup extra-virgin olive oil
1 tablespoon apple cider vinegar
¼ teaspoon sea salt, plus more as needed
Pinch of freshly ground black pepper
3 heads romaine lettuce, halved lengthwise
   through the core
3 endives, halved lengthwise through
   the core

Prepare a grill for high, direct heat, or heat a cast-iron skillet or grill pan on the stovetop over high heat.

In a medium bowl, whisk together the herbs, olive oil, vinegar, salt, and pepper.

Paint the romaine and endive halves all over with the vinaigrette.

Grill the romaine and endive until lightly browned on both sides, 4 to 5 minutes, turning halfway through.

Serve immediately. You can either serve the hearts whole for eating with a knife and fork, or chop them and toss them in a bowl as a salad.

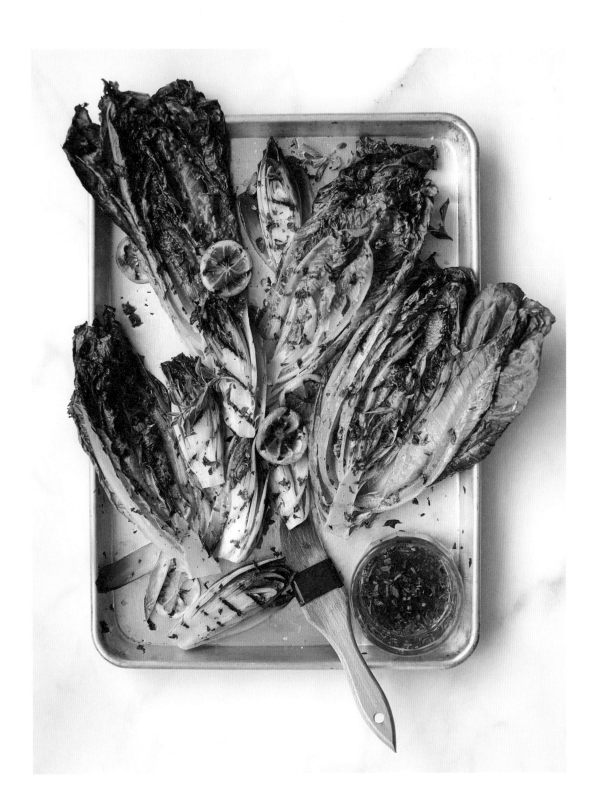

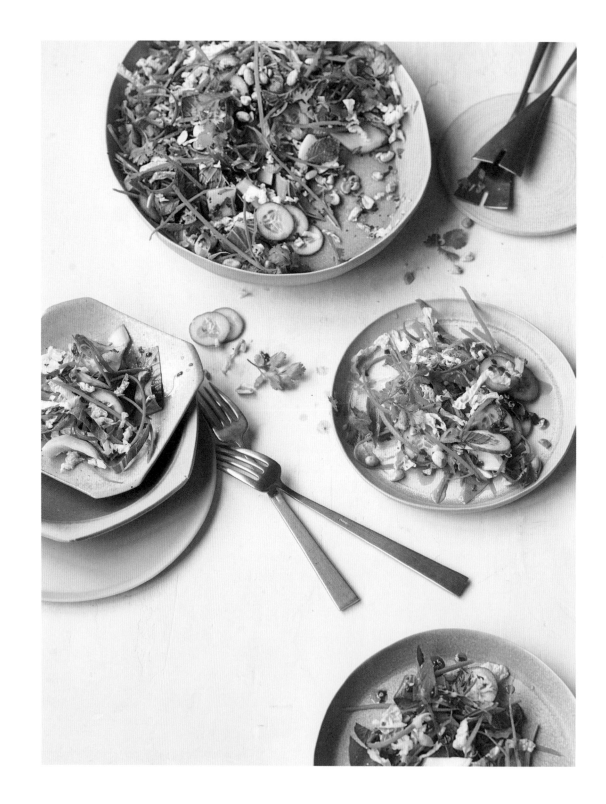

◇

CRUNCHITY VIETNAMESE SALAD

The unusual star ingredient of this salad is bok choy. Bok choy is chock-full of vitamins (A, C, and K) and minerals (calcium, magnesium, potassium, manganese, and iron), and I'm always trying to eat more of this super veggie. This salad is crisp and flavorful, bursting with fresh herbs and lime. Pair it with grilled shrimp, tofu, or fish for a light dinner. You can also add in rice or quinoa for a heartier meal.

serves about 8

Juice of 3 limes

1 tablespoon toasted sesame oil

1½ tablespoons rice vinegar

3 tablespoons tamari or coconut aminos

1 to 2 teaspoons red pepper flakes

Sea salt and freshly ground black pepper

1 large bok choy, thinly sliced

½ small napa cabbage, thinly sliced

1 carrot, thinly sliced

1 cucumber, thinly sliced into rounds (if using a regular cucumber, you'll want to peel the thick skin; Persian-style smaller cucumbers are fine with the skin on)

Leaves from ½ bunch cilantro, chopped

3 tablespoons chopped fresh mint leaves

3 scallions, thinly sliced

¼ cup crushed peanuts, for garnish (optional)

In small bowl, whisk together the lime juice, sesame oil, vinegar, tamari, red pepper flakes, and salt and black pepper to taste.

In a large salad bowl, combine the bok choy, cabbage, carrot, cucumber, cilantro, mint, and scallions and toss to combine.

Add the dressing and toss gently to coat the salad. Garnish with the peanuts, if desired, and serve.

tip

HAVE TROUBLE DIGESTING RAW VEGGIES? YOU CAN TOSS THIS SALAD IN A SKILLET FOR A FEW MINUTES WITH THE DRESSING—IT TASTES GREAT EITHER WAY!

⬦

HEALING GREENS SOUP

This soup is like rehab for your gut and waistline, which is why it's one of the recipes I use in my Good Gut Reset (chapter four). Loaded with good-for-you (and naturally slimming) ingredients plus tons of dark leafy greens, this soup will leave you feeling deeply nourished. You can sip it between meals as a snack, or have a bowl with a poached egg for a more complete reset-style meal.

---

serves 2 to 4

2 to 4 garlic cloves, minced

1 (1-inch) piece fresh ginger, grated

2 bunches dark leafy greens, such as
   spinach, watercress, kale, mustard
   greens, and/or collard greens, chopped

2 to 3 scallions, chopped (optional)

1 yellow onion, chopped

3 tablespoons organic miso paste

Sea salt and freshly ground black pepper

A sprinkle of cayenne pepper

Juice of ½ lemon (about 2 tablespoons)

Fresh herbs, for garnish (optional)

In a medium to large pot, combine the garlic, ginger, and 3 cups water and bring to a boil.

Add the greens and reduce the heat to maintain a simmer.

Add the scallions (if using) and onion and cook for a minute or two, until the greens are tender. You may also need to add additional liquid to generously cover the vegetables. Remove the soup from the heat.

In a small bowl, combine the miso paste with a small amount of the soup broth. Combine thoroughly with a fork and then add the miso mixture to the pot (do not return the pot to the heat).

Season with sea salt, black pepper, cayenne pepper, and lemon juice. Serve as is, or blend the soup directly in the pot with an immersion blender until smooth. You can also garnish with fresh herbs.

◇

SPICED
CARROT
SOUP

Blended veggie soups are one of my top gut-friendly, weight loss foods, and also one of my favorite healthy comfort foods in general. Warm soups are both super satisfying and easy on your belly. This recipe highlights some of my favorite naturally sweet root vegetables, which can help curb sugar cravings.

---

serves 4 to 6

3 tablespoons olive or coconut oil

1 large onion, quartered

½ teaspoon sea salt, plus more for
   seasoning

Freshly ground black pepper

2 garlic cloves, minced

2 tablespoons grated fresh turmeric,
   or 1½ teaspoons ground turmeric

1 tablespoon grated fresh ginger,
   or 1 teaspoon ground ginger

8 to 10 carrots, chopped into chunks

3 parsnips, peeled and chopped into chunks

¼ teaspoon ground cinnamon

2 cups bone broth or broth of your choice

OPTIONAL GARNISHES

Chopped hazelnuts, toasted

Spiced Chickpeas (see page 107)

Fresh thyme leaves

In a large pot, heat 2 tablespoons of the oil over medium heat. Add the onion, season with a little salt and pepper, and cook, stirring, until translucent, about 7 minutes.

Add the remaining 1 tablespoon oil, the garlic, turmeric, and ginger, and reduce the heat to low. Season with pepper and cook until the garlic is browned.

Add the carrots, parsnips, cinnamon, and salt. Add the bone broth and 2 cups water (if you do not have bone broth, you can use all water) and bring to a boil. Reduce the heat to maintain a simmer and cook for 20 minutes.

Blend the soup directly in the pot with an immersion blender until smooth (or transfer to a regular blender and carefully puree until smooth—be careful when blending hot liquids).

Ladle or pour into bowls. Top with toasted hazelnuts, spiced chickpeas, and/or fresh thyme.

◇

NOT-YOUR-GRANDMOTHER'S BORSCHT

My husband wouldn't go near borscht, until he tried this. I'm of eastern European descent and grew up on the stuff (and love it!), but I understand that not everyone feels the same. It's an acquired taste. This version is more like a veggie soup with tons of beets and lentils, but it has that sour-savory thing going on that's so irresistible with classic borscht. Added bonus: Beets are gut- and hormone-balancing.

serves 6 to 8

¼ cup avocado or olive oil

½ onion, diced

2 or 3 garlic cloves, minced

2 celery stalks, chopped

Sea salt and freshly ground black pepper

3 or 4 large beets, chopped (about 5 cups)

2 potatoes, chopped

½ head red cabbage, shredded

Leaves from 4 sprigs thyme

4 bay leaves

1 teaspoon caraway seeds

½ cup lentils (black, brown, or green all work)

¾ cup fresh dill, chopped

Juice of 1 lemon (about 4 tablespoons)

In a large pot, heat the oil over medium heat. Add the onion, garlic, and celery and season generously with salt and pepper. Cook for 5 to 7 minutes, stirring occasionally.

Add the beets, potatoes, and cabbage, season with salt and pepper again, and cook, stirring, for another 5 to 7 minutes.

Add the thyme, bay leaves, caraway seeds, lentils, and water to cover (7 to 8 cups). Bring to a boil, then reduce the heat to maintain a simmer, cover, and cook for about 1 hour, until the lentils are tender and potatoes and beets are easily pierced with a fork. Taste and add more salt and pepper if needed.

Stir in the dill and lemon juice and serve.

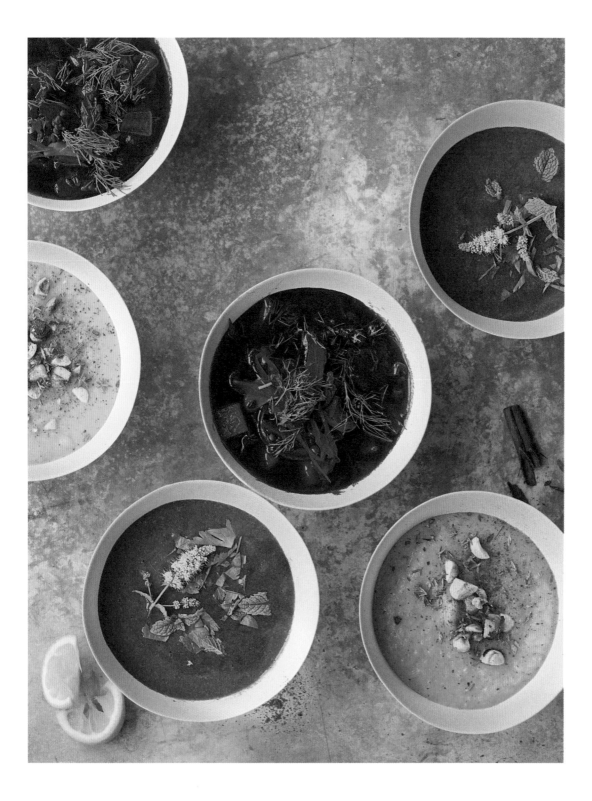

◇

PHO BONE BROTH

This is a fun spin on bone broth, the soup that helps heal your gut lining. Your gut lining works as a barrier between your digestive tract and the rest of your body. If the lining is compromised by poor food choices, stress, or environmental toxins, bad bacteria and undigested food may leak from your gut into your body and cause inflammation. Bone broth is my secret weapon, and this pho version is extra delicious.

---

makes about 8 cups

2 marrow bones, cut in half lengthwise (ask your butcher to do this for you)

Sea salt

2 lemongrass stalks

1 cinnamon stick

1 tablespoon coriander seeds

1 tablespoon fennel seeds

1 green cardamom pod

1 (1-inch) piece fresh ginger, sliced

2 scallions, cut into large pieces, plus sliced scallions for garnish

Sliced Thai red chiles, for garnish (optional)

tip

LOOKING FOR SOME BASIC BONE BROTH RECIPES? HEAD TO ROBYNYOUKILIS.COM/BOOKS!

Preheat the oven to 400°F. Place the bones on a baking sheet, cut-side up, and sprinkle with salt. Bake for 15 minutes, or until the marrow is bubbling. Scoop out the marrow and reserve it for later use (it's great on toast!). Put the bones in a large pot.

Peel away the tough outer layers of the lemongrass stalks to reveal the pale inner cores and trim the bottoms with a sharp knife. Crush the stems with the flat side of a knife to release the flavor. Add the lemongrass to the pot with the marrow bones.

Add the cinnamon stick, coriander, fennel, cardamom, ginger, scallions, and 10 cups water. Bring to a boil.

Reduce the heat to maintain a simmer, cover, and cook for at least 4 hours, and up to 8 hours. Strain the broth and discard the bones and veggies. I'll sometimes push the veggies, pressing with the back of a spoon to extract all the liquid.

Ladle some bone broth into a bowl or mug and garnish with scallions and/or Thai chiles when you're ready to drink! Let the remaining broth cool to room temperature and store in an airtight container in the fridge for up to 5 days or in the freezer for up to 1 year.

◇

HEARTY
WINTER STEW

This stew is the ideal all-in-one cold weather meal. Collard greens are full of iron, protein, and fiber, as well as a number of vitamins and minerals. You can use a veggie, chicken, turkey, or pork sausage in this recipe—they all turn out yummy!

---

serves 6

1 pound any kind of Italian sausage,
    removed from casing and crumbled or
    sliced into small bite-size pieces
Olive oil or ghee for cooking, if needed
1 onion, diced
2 celery stalks, diced
2 carrots, diced
2 garlic cloves, minced
Sea salt and freshly ground black pepper
1 (28-ounce) can crushed tomatoes
1 tablespoon tomato paste
1 bunch collard greens or any kale variety,
    stemmed, leaves thinly sliced

In a large pot, brown the sausage over medium heat, 7 to 8 minutes, then remove and set aside on a plate.

If your pan is dry after cooking your sausage, add a tablespoon or two of oil or ghee. Add the onion, celery, carrots, and garlic to the pot, season with salt and pepper, and cook, stirring, until softened, 8 to 10 minutes.

Return the sausage and any juices from the plate to the pot.

Add the crushed tomatoes and tomato paste and season with a bit more salt.

Add 1 to 2 cups water and bring to a simmer. Cover and simmer for 20 minutes.

Add the collards and cook until they are wilted, about 5 minutes more.

Serve and enjoy.

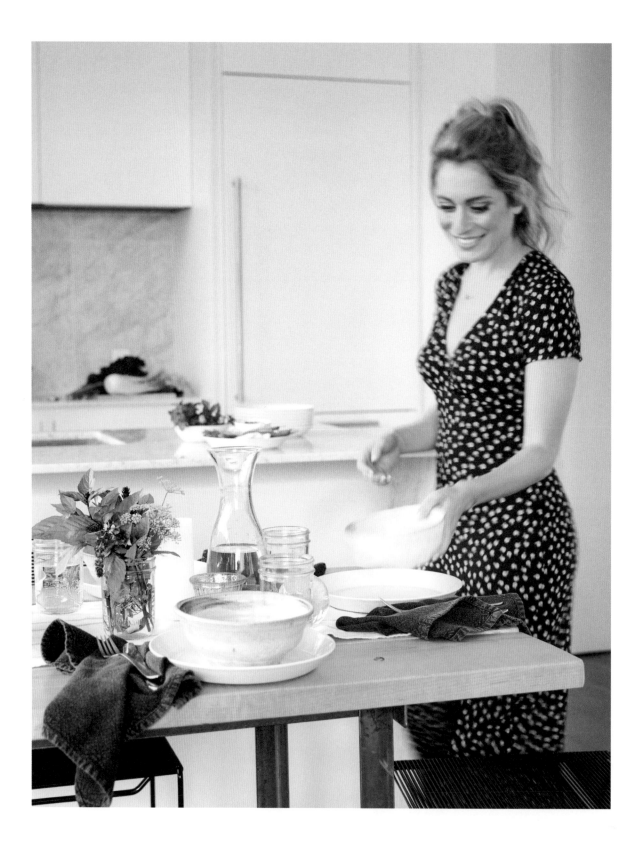

THE
MAIN EVENT

◇

CLASSIC LAMB TAGINE

When I eat out, I usually go for Moroccan food. It's so flavorful and usually pretty healthy. One of the most popular dishes at my local Moroccan spot is a tagine. It gets its name from the traditional earthen vessel in which the food is cooked. Don't worry—you won't need to go out and buy a new pot; my variation can be baked in any oven-safe dish or a slow cooker. Translation? You throw everything together in the morning and have an awesome dinner ready at the end of the day.

---

serves 4

2 pounds lamb stew meat, cut into cubes

Sea salt and freshly ground black pepper

1 onion, chopped

6 to 8 carrots, chopped

1 (15-ounce) can chickpeas, rinsed and
   drained (optional)

2 garlic cloves, minced

2 tablespoons ground ginger

2 tablespoons ground cumin

2 tablespoons paprika

2 tablespoons onion powder

2 tablespoons garlic powder

½ cup dried apricots, halved

¾ cup pitted prunes

¼ cup fresh parsley, chopped,
   for garnish (optional)

Herbed Quinoa Pilaf (page 158) or Good Gut
   Green Rice (page 159), for serving

TO COOK IN A SLOW COOKER:
Combine all the ingredients except the parsley in a 6-quart slow cooker and add 2 to 3 cups of water to generously cover. Cover and cook on high for 4 to 5 hours or low for 7 hours.

TO COOK ON THE STOVETOP:
Pat the lamb dry and season it with salt and pepper. Heat a large saucepan over medium heat. Add the lamb and cook until browned on all sides, about 10 minutes. Transfer the meat to a plate and set aside.

Put the onion and a dash of salt in the same pan and cook until translucent, 5 to 7 minutes.

Add the chickpeas, if using, the carrots, garlic, spices, apricots, and prunes and cook, stirring, for 3 minutes more.

Return the meat to the pot and add 2 to 3 cups water to generously cover. Bring to a boil, then reduce the heat to maintain a simmer, and cook uncovered for 1 hour.

Garnish with the parsley and serve with herbed quinoa pilaf or green rice.

◇

SURF-OR-TURF FAJITAS

TGI Fridays sizzling fajitas were my favorite thing growing up. The "adult me" still loves this DIY-style meal—anytime I get to assemble my plate exactly the way I want it, I'm a happy gal. For this reason, homemade fajitas easily fit the Good Gut Rule of Five—you can load up on the veggies, protein, and healthy fats, the ideal plate combo. Plus, I find this type of dish forces me sloooow down, which is a key part of my approach to healthy weight loss.

---

serves 8 to 10

3 tablespoons tamari or coconut aminos

Juice of 2 limes

2 tablespoons olive oil, plus more for
   cooking

2 tablespoons coconut sugar

1 tablespoon plus ½ teaspoon ground cumin

4 garlic cloves, crushed

1½ pounds skirt steak or peeled
   and deveined shrimp

1 red onion, sliced

3 bell peppers, not green, sliced

½ teaspoon chili powder

1 teaspoon dried oregano

1 teaspoon sea salt

¼ teaspoon cayenne pepper

1 beefsteak tomato, diced

Guacamole (store-bought is okay)

Plain yogurt, for serving

Fresh herbs, chopped, for serving

In a large bowl, combine the tamari, lime juice, 2 tablespoons olive oil, coconut sugar, 1 tablespoon of the cumin, and the garlic.

Add the steak or shrimp to the bowl, cover, and marinate in the refrigerator. If using steak, let sit for 1 to 2 hours. If using shrimp, you'll only want to let it marinate for 10 to 15 minutes.

In a large skillet, heat olive oil over medium heat. Add the onion and cook, stirring, for 5 minutes. Add the bell peppers, chili powder, oregano, salt, the remaining cumin, and the cayenne and cook for 3 minutes more.

Add the steak or shrimp and as much of the marinade as you'd like and cook, stirring, until the steak is cooked to your liking or the shrimp are pink and opaque. If using steak, remove it from the pan and let it rest for a few minutes, then slice it into thin strips across the grain.

Serve in tortillas or over rice (or cauliflower rice) or greens. Top with the tomato, guac, a dollop of yogurt, and herbs.

◇

ROCKSTAR VEGGIE BURGERS

I've been on the hunt for a good homemade veggie burger recipe for years. I shared a black bean burger variation in my first book, but I wanted to come up with a bean-free option, since legumes can be difficult for a lot of people to digest. These cauliflower–sweet potato burgers are loaded with digestion-boosting herbs and spices. Plus they pack in a ton of veggies. Serve them on a burger bun of choice, atop a salad, or on a Good Gut Rule of Five bowl.

makes 6 burgers

QUICK-PICKLED ONIONS

1 medium red onion, thinly sliced

¾ cup red wine vinegar
  or apple cider vinegar

BURGERS

Coconut or avocado oil spray, if needed

1 head cauliflower, cored and chopped

4 small sweet potatoes,
  peeled and chopped

1 tablespoon coconut oil, melted

½ teaspoon sea salt, plus more as needed

Freshly ground black pepper

¼ cup fresh cilantro, finely chopped

½ teaspoon ground cumin

Juice of ½ lime

½ teaspoon chili powder

½ teaspoon garlic powder

Smashed avocado, for topping

Cover the onion with the vinegar and let sit for at least 15 minutes, then drain. Preheat the oven to 425ºF. Line a baking sheet with parchment paper or spray with coconut or avocado oil spray. In a large bowl, toss the cauliflower, sweet potatoes, and coconut oil to coat, then transfer to the baking sheet, season with the salt and pepper, and roast for about 30 minutes, until golden brown. Let cool slightly.

Transfer the roasted cauliflower and sweet potatoes to a food processor and pulse until mostly smooth (or transfer to a bowl and mash with a fork). Transfer to a bowl (if necessary) and add the cilantro, cumin, lime juice, chili powder, and garlic powder. Mix to incorporate.

Form the mixture into patties about ½ inch thick and place them on the baking sheet you used for the vegetables. Bake for 30 minutes, flipping the burgers once halfway through. You may need to use two spatulas when flipping these, as they can be delicate. Finish the burgers by broiling on high for 5 to 10 minutes.

Top burgers with smashed avocado and some quick-pickled onions.

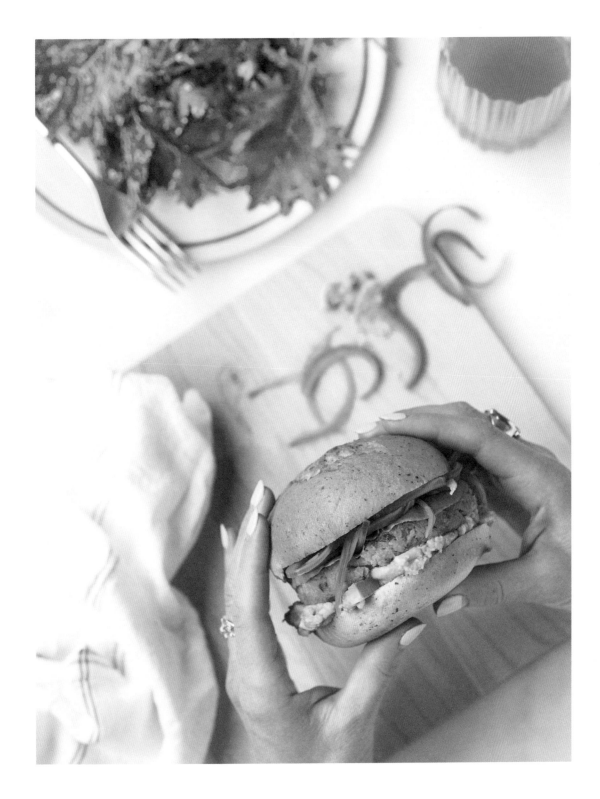

◇

THE SIMPLEST SALMON

My sweet mother-in-law is an amazing cook, and I always turn to her for easy fish recipes that wow. Whether you're throwing together a 20-minute weeknight meal or want to impress guests at a dinner party without spending hours in the kitchen, this salmon is a go-to. Salmon is a dense source of protein and healthy fat, both key for gut health and weight loss. This pairs beautifully with some simply grilled asparagus and the green rice on page 159.

serves 3 or 4

2 tablespoons room-temperature or melted
   ghee or butter
1 pound skin-on salmon fillet
Sea salt and freshly ground black pepper
½ cup sliced almonds, very lightly toasted
Drizzle of raw honey (optional)

Preheat the oven to 400°F. Use some of the ghee or butter to grease a large baking dish.

Put the salmon in the baking dish. Rub the rest of the ghee or butter on top of the salmon and season generously with salt and pepper. Cover it with the toasted almonds.

Bake for 12 minutes. Remove from the oven and, if using, drizzle the honey over the entire fillet. Return to the oven and bake for another 3 to 8 minutes (depending on thickness of the fish). Check for doneness by flaking with a fork—the salmon should break but not fall apart. The salmon will continue to cook a little on its own after you remove it from the oven, so you don't want it to dry out. Serve and eat!

VEGGIE-PACKED MEATBALLS

Meatballs are the ultimate meal prep item—whether you're making turkey, lamb, fish (yes, fish works great here!), or beef, these can be used in so many ways. Pair them with a salad and prepped roasted root veggies, and you have a meal in 15 minutes or less. Bonus: This take on the classic has way more veggies (are you noticing a trend here?) without compromising the distinctive Italian flavor profile.

---

serves 4 to 6

Oil, for greasing (optional)

1 pound ground beef, turkey, chicken, pork, or fish

3½ cups grated veggies, such as zucchini, carrot, onion, and fennel

1 teaspoon sea salt

2 large eggs

2 tablespoons Italian seasoning (see Note)

Preheat the oven to 350°F. Line a rimmed baking sheet with parchment paper or grease with oil.

Combine all the ingredients in a bowl and mix until well incorporated.

Form the meat mixture into roughly 2-inch balls and arrange them on the prepared baking sheet.

Bake for 15 to 20 minutes, until well browned.

note

IN PLACE OF THE ITALIAN SEASONING; YOU CAN MAKE YOUR OWN BLEND BY COMBINING CHOPPED FRESH ROSEMARY, FRESH THYME LEAVES, MINCED GARLIC, FRESHLY GROUND BLACK PEPPER, AND RED PEPPER FLAKES TO TOTAL 3 TABLESPOONS.

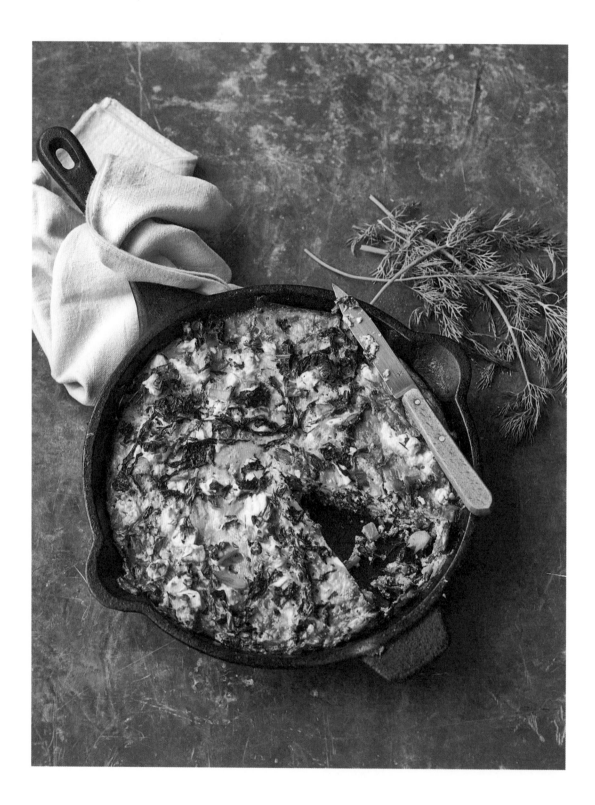

KALE SKILLET SPANAKOPITA

◇

Yes, I said kale, and yes, I said spanakopita. This version of the classic is adapted from the amazing Doris Choi's recipe and skips the phyllo dough in favor of tons of kale and lots of fresh herbs and spices. A cast-iron skillet works best here as it's naturally nonstick and stays hotter than other pots and pans. Plus, cooking with cast iron adds iron (a nutrient many of us are low or deficient in) to your dish.

---

serves about 6

1 teaspoon unsalted butter, olive oil, or coconut oil

3 garlic cloves, minced

½ onion, chopped

1 fennel bulb, cored and chopped

½ teaspoon sea salt

¼ teaspoon freshly ground black pepper

5 large eggs

2 scallions, chopped

½ cup fresh dill, chopped

½ cup fresh parsley, chopped

4 to 6 ounces feta cheese, crumbled

1 bunch kale, stemmed and finely chopped

Preheat the oven to 350°F.

In a large cast-iron skillet, melt the butter over medium heat. Add the garlic, onion, and fennel, season with the salt and pepper, and cook, stirring, for 5 to 7 minutes.

In a large bowl, whisk together the eggs, scallions, dill, parsley, and feta. Set aside.

Add the chopped kale to the vegetables and onions in the skillet and continue cooking, stirring, for 5 minutes, or until the kale has wilted.

Slowly add the vegetable mixture to the bowl with the egg mixture, stir to combine, and transfer everything back to the skillet.

Put the skillet in the oven and bake for 15 to 25 minutes. Your spanakopita is done when the center has set and the edges begin to brown. Serve immediately or let cool and store in an airtight container in the refrigerator for meals throughout the week.

tip

THIS RECIPE REHEATS BEAUTIFULLY AND MAKES A PERFECT PARTY APPETIZER, BREAKFAST, LUNCH, DINNER, OR SNACK— IT'S TRULY MULTIPURPOSE.

◇

AMAZING MARBELLA, TWO WAYS

Growing up, I would thumb through my mom's cookbook collection and find one of my favorites, The Silver Palate Cookbook by Julee Rosso and Sheila Lukins. As an incredible entertainer, then and now, my mom would often look here for inspiration. Chicken Marbella is one of the most famous dishes from that book, with its special combo of sweet prunes with briny capers and olives. This adaptation works great for batch cooking or for entertaining.

serves 6 to 8

1 to 2 chickens (about 5 pounds in total),
    quartered, or 2 packages (about 1½
    pounds) firm tofu
¼ cup olive oil
¼ cup apple cider vinegar
½ cup pitted prunes
¼ cup pitted Spanish green olives
¼ cup capers in brine, drained
3 bay leaves
1 head garlic, cloves separated and
    smashed or minced
¼ cup fresh oregano, chopped,
    or 2 tablespoons dried
1 teaspoon sea salt
Pinch of freshly ground black pepper
1 to 2 tablespoons coconut sugar
½ cup white wine
1 to 2 tablespoons chopped fresh parsley

If using chicken, pat the pieces dry and place them in a large bowl. If using tofu, drain the packages and wrap the tofu blocks in paper towels. Put them in a roasting pan and place a small plate on top of each. Place a weight (a book, a heavy bowl, a can of tomatoes, etc.) on top of each plate to apply pressure. Set aside for at least 1 hour.

In a large bowl, combine the olive oil, vinegar, prunes, olives, capers, bay leaves, garlic, oregano, salt, and pepper. Add the chicken or tofu to the mixture. Cover with plastic wrap and marinate in the refrigerator for at least 6 hours and up to 24 hours.

When you're ready to bake, preheat the oven to 350°F.

Transfer the chicken or tofu to a roasting pan and pour the marinade over the top. Sprinkle with the coconut sugar and top with the wine.

Bake for 1 to 1½ hours. The chicken is done when thigh pieces yield clear golden juices (not pink) when pricked with a fork. The tofu is done when the top begins to brown.

Garnish with the parsley before serving.

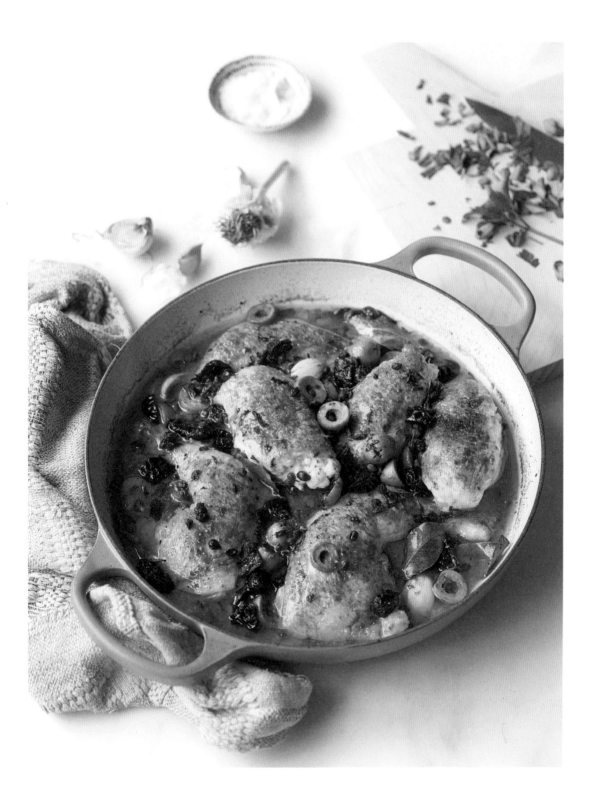

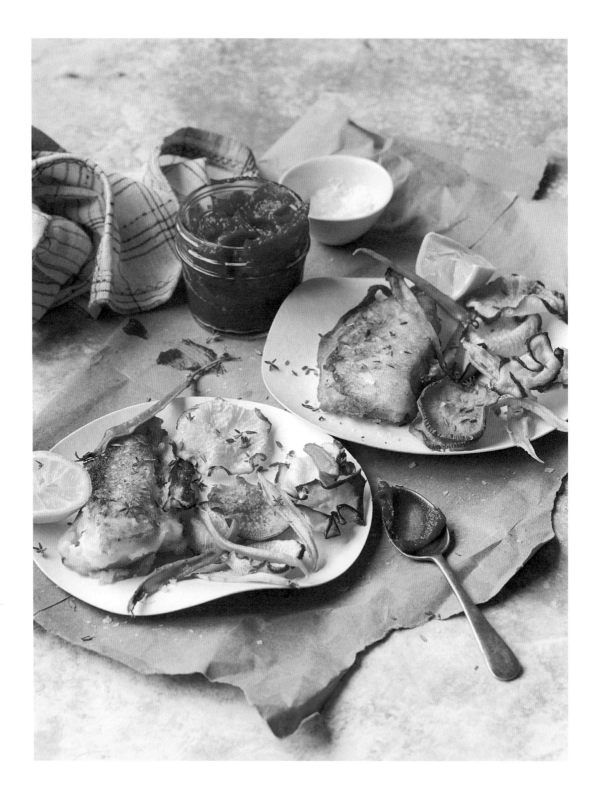

◇

'BOOCH-BATTERED FISH AND CHIPS

Fish and chips is a classic comfort meal, but not exactly the most weight-loss friendly dish. Solution? Use kombucha and a gluten-free flour, and pan-fry instead of deep-frying. If you want a fun, family-friendly dinner, make this tonight. Serve with my Root Veggie Chips and Amped-Up Ketchup (page 132).

---

serves 3

1 pound cod, flounder, or hake, cut into large "fingers"

Pinch of sea salt, plus more for seasoning

8 to 10 ounces plain kombucha

1 teaspoon baking powder

1 ½ cups brown or white rice flour

3 tablespoons coconut oil

Vinegar of your choice or fresh lemon juice

Fresh thyme leaves, for serving

Season the fish with salt.

In a bowl, combine the kombucha, baking powder, salt, and flour.

In a medium nonstick skillet, melt the coconut oil over medium heat. Test the oil by dropping a bit of batter into the pan; if it sizzles, you're ready to sear.

Dip the fish "fingers" in the batter, shake off any excess, and carefully place in the hot oil. Do not crowd the pan.

Cook the fish for 2 to 3 minutes on each side, until lightly browned. Repeat with the remaining fish.

Enjoy with your favorite vinegar or a squeeze of lemon and a sprinkle of thyme leaves.

AMPED-UP KETCHUP

Serves 6 to 8

1 (7-ounce) jar organic tomato paste

2 to 3 tablespoons pure maple syrup

1 tablespoon sauerkraut juice (from a jar or

container of prepared sauerkraut)

Pinch of cayenne pepper

¾ teaspoon sea salt

1 small garlic clove, minced

Combine all the ingredients in a bowl and mix well.

Transfer the ketchup to a jar that leaves a little room for expansion at the top and seal. Set aside to ferment at room temperature for a minimum of 24 hours and up to 3 days. You can taste the ketchup after the first 24 hours and see if it's tangy enough for your taste buds. If not, let it keep fermenting and unscrew the lid once a day to let gas escape.

When it's fermented to your liking, transfer the jar to the fridge. The ketchup will keep for up to 3 weeks.

ROOT VEGGIE CHIPS

serves 4 to 6
(or 2, if you really like them!) as a side

2 golden beets, peeled and thinly sliced

1 small rutabaga or jicama, peeled and thinly sliced

1 to 2 tablespoons avocado oil or coconut oil

Sea salt and freshly ground black pepper

Preheat the oven to 225°F.

Combine the root veggies in a large bowl and toss with the avocado oil.

Arrange the veggies on a baking sheet in a single layer (use another baking sheet if you need to so that the veggie chips don't overlap).

Bake for 1 to 1½ hours, until browned and some of the edges start to curl.

Remove from the oven and season with salt and pepper.

◇

SPAGHETTI SQUASH BOLOGNESE

When I'm craving pasta, I often find that what I really want is heaps of tomato sauce, so I'll make spaghetti squash in the style of classic Bolognese. I switch the ratio so there's about twice as much veggies as meat, and suddenly, what used to be a classic "diet no-no" food becomes a comforting weight loss–friendly weeknight dinner.

serves 8

Coconut oil

1 spaghetti squash, halved

Sea salt and freshly ground black pepper

2 tablespoons extra-virgin olive oil

1 onion, chopped

2 garlic cloves, chopped

Leaves from 2 sprigs rosemary, finely
   chopped or left whole

3 celery stalks, chopped

3 medium carrots, chopped

1½ pounds ground meat
   (such as turkey, beef or lamb)

1 (28-ounce) can crushed tomatoes

Pinch of red pepper flakes

Preheat the oven to 375°F.

Rub coconut oil on the cut sides of the squash and season with salt and black pepper. Set the squash cut-side down on a baking sheet. Bake for 30 to 45 minutes, until fork-tender. Use a fork to scrape the squash flesh into strands; discard the skin.

In a large skillet, heat the olive oil over medium heat. Add the onion and garlic with a pinch of salt and cook, stirring, until the onion is translucent, about 10 minutes.

Add the rosemary, celery, and carrots, season with a bit more salt and black pepper, and cook, stirring, for 5 minutes more. Add the ground meat and cook until browned, 7 to 10 minutes.

Add the crushed tomatoes and season with salt, black pepper, and the red pepper flakes. Simmer the sauce for 5 to 10 more minutes.

Serve the sauce over the cooked spaghetti squash immediately, or reduce the heat to maintain a simmer, cover, and keep warm for up to 20 minutes before serving.

SPAGHETTI SWITCH UP

VEGETARIAN Swap the meat in the recipe on page 133 for some vegetarian-style meatballs or crumbled tempeh.

PESTO PERFECTION Mix roasted spaghetti squash with 1 to 2 spiralized zuchinni. Toss with pesto and top with sauteed shrimp.

PUT AN EGG ON IT While you're roasting the spaghetti squash, roast a tray of cherry tomatoes tossed in olive oil on a separate pan. Top the squash with the tomatoes, a poached egg, some snipped chives, and black pepper.

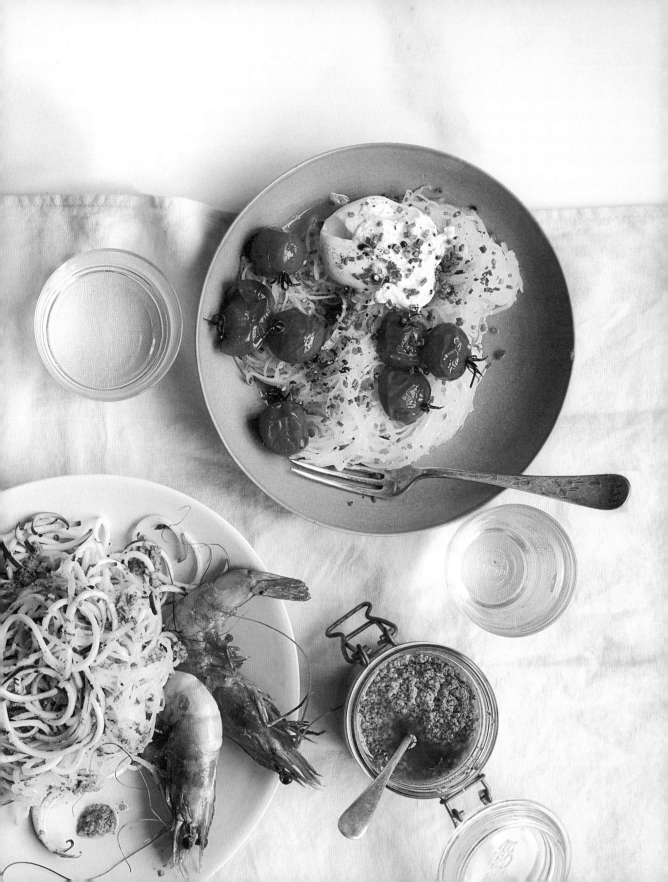

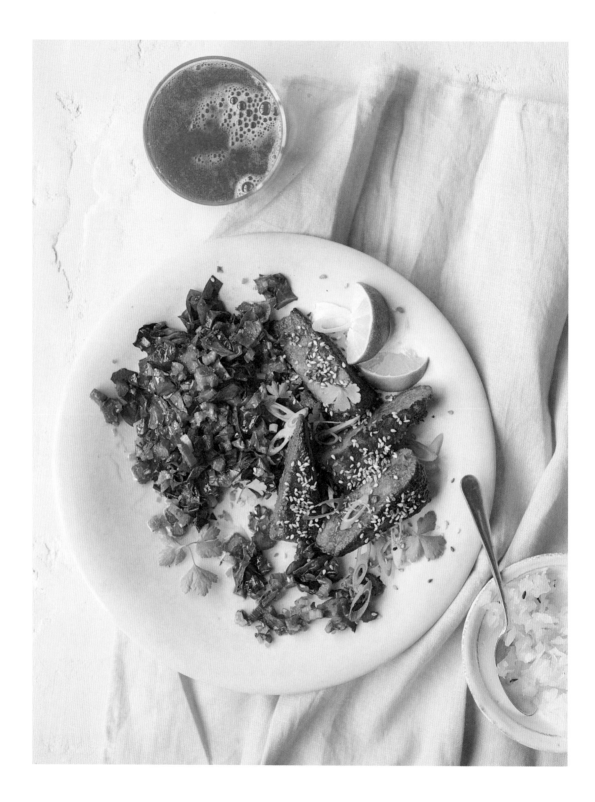

◇

SAVORY SUNFLOWER BUTTER TEMPEH

Tempeh is a weekly staple in my diet, as it's a gut-friendly vegetarian protein. I usually simply sear it in coconut oil and tamari, but when I want to mix it up, I make this version that tastes even better than Chinese takeout. You can add this tempeh to a salad, or serve it with stir-fry veggies and rice (or cauliflower rice!) for a complete meal.

serves 2 to 3

¼ teaspoon red pepper flakes

2 tablespoons toasted sesame oil

2 tablespoons sunflower seed butter
(or almond or peanut butter)

2 tablespoons tamari or coconut aminos

Juice of 1 lime

3 tablespoons pure maple syrup

10 ounces tempeh, cut into 1-inch triangles
or sliced

OPTIONAL GARNISHES

Scallions, sliced

Sesame seeds

Fresh cilantro and/or parsley, chopped

Combine all the ingredients except the tempeh and garnishes in a medium bowl and mix well. Add the tempeh and turn to coat well in the marinade. Cover and marinate in the refrigerator for at least 2 hours and up to overnight (24 hours is great!).

When ready to cook the tempeh, preheat the oven to 375°F. Line a baking sheet with parchment paper.

Spread the tempeh on the prepared baking sheet in an even layer; set the marinade aside.

Bake for 20 to 30 minutes, until the tempeh is golden brown and caramelized. Remove the baking sheet from the oven and brush the tempeh with the reserved marinade.

Garnish as desired and serve.

tip

SUNFLOWER SEED BUTTER IS A NICE
ALLERGEN-FREE SWAP
FOR NUT BUTTERS.

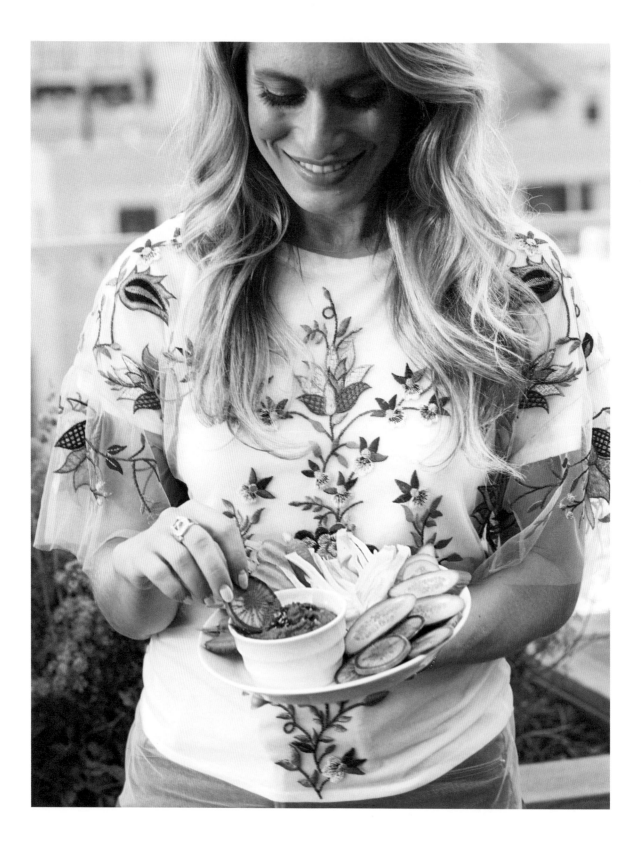

SNACKS, SIDES, AND SHAREABLES

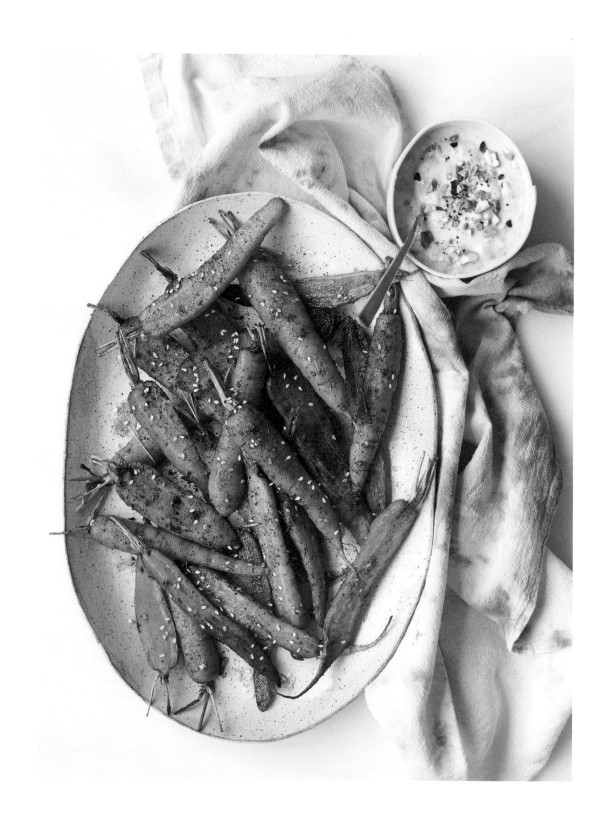

◇

ZA'ATAR-
ROASTED
CARROTS

When I tested these babies, they didn't even make it to the table—my family ate almost all of them off the tray. They were that good. When you roast carrots they become super sweet, almost like candy. When you add savory za'atar spice, nutty pistachios, and aromatic cardamom cream, you have the ultimate side or appetizer.

serves 4

1 pound carrots, cut into sticks
  or halved lengthwise

1 to 2 tablespoons coconut oil, melted

½ teaspoon sea salt

½ teaspoon ground cumin

2 tablespoons za'atar (see Note)

1 small container plain goat's-milk yogurt

1 teaspoon ground cardamom

¼ cup pistachios, chopped

Preheat the oven to 425°F.

In a large bowl, toss the carrots with the coconut oil and place on a rimmed baking sheet

Sprinkle with the salt, cumin, and za'atar.

Roast for 25 to 35 minutes, until browned to your liking.

Meanwhile, in a small bowl, whisk together the yogurt and cardamom.

Garnish the carrots with the cardamom cream and chopped pistachios.

tip

THE SPICED ROASTED CARROTS ARE WONDERFUL EVEN WITHOUT THE PISTACHIOS AND CARDAMOM CREAM, IF YOU ARE SHORT ON TIME OR INGREDIENTS!

note

ZA'ATAR IS A SPICE BLEND MADE WITH THYME, DRIED SUMAC, SESAME SEEDS, AND OFTEN OTHER HERBS AND SPICES. YOU CAN FIND IT AT MIDDLE EASTERN GROCERIES OR ONLINE, OR MAKE YOUR OWN BLEND AT HOME.

◇

RUBY
RED KRAUT

While both red and green cabbage are good for you, red cabbage actually contains twice as much vitamin C and more inflammation-fighting phytonutrients. Red cabbage also has a slightly different flavor which makes this ruby kraut a bit more zippy than a more traditional recipe.

---

makes about 4 cups

1 large head red cabbage,
   2 outer leaves removed and reserved,
   remainder finely shredded
1 tablespoon sea salt or Himalayan pink
   salt, plus more if needed
1 medium beet, shredded
Filtered water

In a large bowl, mix the shredded cabbage and salt by hand until it gets all juicy, with liquid pooling at the bottom of the bowl.

You'll want to spend a bit of time on this! Taste it throughout; it should taste very, very salty. Add the shredded beet and mix again.

Pack the veggies into a quart mason jar. You'll want to stuff the jar with an inch or two of the veggies and pack it tightly down, then add another inch or two and repeat. Liquid should come up and cover the veggies at each stage of the packing and layering. Pack the veggies until you reach the top of the jar, leaving an inch or two of headspace. Make sure the veggies are below the liquid. Add a splash of filtered water if needed to keep them covered (or you may need a smaller jar, depending on quantity of cabbage used).

Fold one of the reserved outer cabbage leaves and place it over the veggies in the jar to further press the veggies below the liquid line. Seal the jar loosely. Leave at room temperature in a cool, dark place to ferment for 1 week or more. "Burp" the kraut every day or two. (To do this, simply unscrew the lid and allow the air to escape, then seal again.) You may need to pack the veggies down with your fist again if they're not covered with liquid.

After about one week, taste the kraut. It should taste sour and slightly salty with a tangy flavor and have a nice but strong aroma. If it tastes good, it's good. If it tastes bad, you may need to scrape off the top layer and discard it, then see if the kraut tastes yummy beneath the liquid. Ferment for as long as your heart desires. I find that anywhere between 10 days and 1 month tastes great (but you can let some ferments go a year or more!). Once the taste is to your liking, seal the jar tightly and store in the fridge for months.

PLANTAIN CHIPS

Plantains are an underused source of prebiotic fiber (that's the fiber that feeds those good probiotic bugs in your gut). You can serve these with hummus (like my Beet Hummus on page 148), black bean dip, or eat 'em straight up.

serves 4

2 plantains (green or yellow; green will be starchier, while yellow will be sweeter), thinly sliced on a mandoline into strips or rounds

2 teaspoons coconut oil or coconut oil spray
1 teaspoon sea salt
Squeeze of fresh lime juice

Preheat the oven to 375°F. Line a baking sheet with parchment paper.

Rub the sliced plantains with coconut oil or spray with coconut oil spray. Arrange them on the prepared baking sheet and sprinkle with the salt. Roast for 15 to 20 minutes.

Squeeze lime juice over the top before serving.

SUPERFOOD SEAWEED CHIPS

If there was ever a yummy superfood snack, this is it. Seaweed is high in natural minerals including folate, calcium, magnesium, zinc, iron, selenium, and iodine. Iodine is crucial for proper thyroid function and metabolism.

serves 1 or 2

1 teaspoon coconut oil
1 package whole leaf dulse

Sea salt

In a large skillet, melt the coconut oil over medium heat.

Add the dulse and cook until crisp, about 5 minutes.

Finish with a sprinkle of sea salt and eat!

tip

DULSE IS A BURGUNDY-COLORED SEAWEED THAT'S USUALLY SOLD DRIED.

◇

PRETTY-IN-PINK FERMENTED RADISHES

Brined cut or whole veggies are some of the easiest fermented foods to make, and they taste seriously gourmet. These fermented radishes are awesome in salads, or as part of a Go with Your Gut Rule of Five plate. If you've been on the fence about fermenting your own veggies, start here.

makes about 1 ½ cups

3 bunches radishes, thinly sliced

1 teaspoon pink peppercorns

¾ cup fresh dill, chopped

1 teaspoon sea salt

Filtered water

Kale, cabbage, or collard leaf

Combine the radishes, peppercorns, dill, and salt in a large bowl. Squish by hand until the radishes have released their liquid.

Transfer the radish mixture to a 12-ounce mason jar and press down so the liquid covers the radishes. If it does not cover the radishes, add filtered water as needed.

Place the kale leaf over the radishes so they stay submerged.

Seal loosely and set aside in a cool, dark place to ferment. "Burp" the radishes once a day for the first 3 days.

Ferment the radishes for 1 to 3 weeks. Begin tasting after 1 week. When they are fermented to your liking, move them to the fridge. They will keep in the fridge for up to 6 months.

note

YOU'LL WANT TO USE A FRESH, CLEAN FORK EVERY TIME YOU SCOOP RADISHES FROM THE JAR. THIS KEEPS THE UNIQUE BACTERIA IN YOUR MOUTH FROM MIXING AND MULTIPLYING IN YOUR JAR.

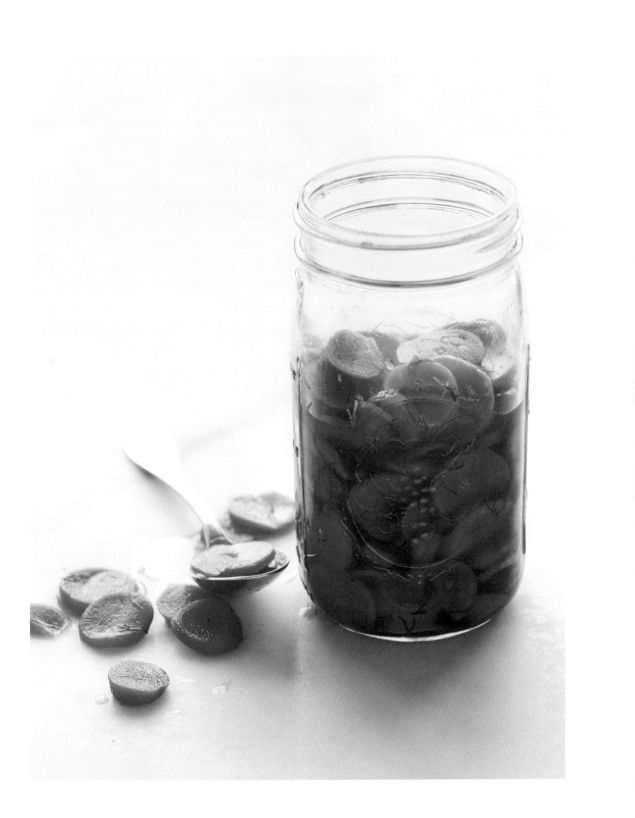

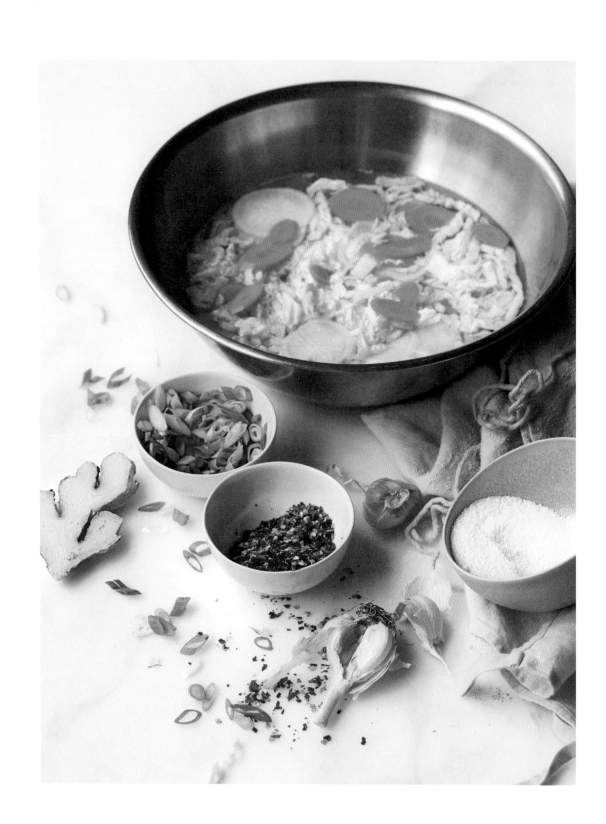

◇

EASY
KIMCHI

Add a couple of spoonfuls of this spicy and exotic ferment to your next stir-fry or Bibimbap Breakfast Bowl (page 78), or mix some into a lunchtime salad for a serious kick of flavor. The best part about making your own kimchi is that you can adjust the level of spiciness to your liking by using more or less (like me!) red pepper flakes.

---

makes about 8 cups

1 napa cabbage, outer leaves removed and
   reserved, remainder sliced
2 carrots, cut into ribbons or thinly sliced
   on an angle
1 daikon radish (about 6 inches), thinly sliced
Filtered water
1 tablespoon sea salt
1 bunch scallions, sliced
4 garlic cloves, thinly sliced
1 (1-inch) piece fresh ginger, peeled and grated
1 to 3 teaspoons red pepper flakes

note

TO BURP YOUR KIMCHI, SIMPLY UNSCREW
THE LID AND ALLOW THE AIR TO ESCAPE,
THEN SEAL AGAIN.

Place the sliced cabbage, carrots, and daikon in a large bowl. Add filtered water to cover, stir in the salt, and cover with a tea towel or plastic wrap. Let sit at room temperature for 24 to 48 hours.

Then pour off most of the water; you want the vegetables to still be wet, but not drowning in liquid. Add the scallions, garlic, ginger, and 1 teaspoon of the red pepper flakes and mix together. Taste and add up to 2 teaspoons more red pepper flakes for more kick.

Transfer the vegetable mixture into a half-gallon-size mason jar or two quart jars and push down to immerse the veggies in the liquid. Add filtered water, if needed, to cover the veggies and top with one of the reserved cabbage leaves.

Seal the jar loosely and set aside in a cool, dark place to ferment. "Burp" the kimchi daily for the first week and once every few days thereafter.

Ferment for 1 to 4 weeks. You can taste the kimchi every few days as it ferments. When the flavor is to your liking, seal the jar and store in the fridge for up to 6 months.

◇

BEAUTIFUL BEET HUMMUS

This beet version of classic hummus is bright and beautiful, and a fun way to get kids (or anyone) to eat more veggies. Who wouldn't want to eat cucumber rounds or celery sticks dipped in something hot pink? It's equally delicious spread on toast, or added to salads and bowl meals instead of a dressing.

makes about 2 cups

1 small beet (you can also purchase
   pre-cooked beets for a shortcut)
1 (15-ounce) can chickpeas,
   drained and rinsed
Juice of 1 lemon
1 teaspoon sea salt
Pinch of freshly ground black pepper
Pinch of cayenne pepper
2 garlic cloves, minced
2 tablespoons tahini
¼ cup extra-virgin olive oil,
   plus more for drizzling
1 tablespoon ground cumin
Chopped fresh parsley, for garnish
Crudités, bread, or crackers, for serving

Preheat the oven to 400°F.

Wrap the beet in aluminum foil and place it in a small roasting pan. Roast until fork-tender, about 25 minutes. Let cool, then unwrap, chop, and place in a food processor.

Add the chickpeas, lemon juice, salt, black and cayenne peppers, garlic, tahini, olive oil, and cumin and process until smooth. Taste and add more salt, pepper, or other seasoning if needed.

Spread on a platter or spoon into a bowl, drizzle with olive oil, and garnish with parsley.

Enjoy with crudités or on your favorite crackers or bread!

◇

LOVE
YOUR LIVER
PÂTÉ

In general, organ meats are between 10 and 100 hundred times higher in nutrients than corresponding muscle meats; liver, in particular, is rich in vitamins A, D, E, K, B12, and folic acid, as well as copper and iron. However, liver, like so many other foods, has been slowly phased out of our everyday diets, mostly because these foods aren't fashionable. Give liver a try with this rich pâté recipe.

makes about 2 cups

3 tablespoons ghee

1 garlic clove, minced

1 onion, finely chopped

1 bay leaf

1 sprig fresh thyme

1 sprig fresh rosemary

1 sprig fresh sage

¼ teaspoon sea salt, plus more as needed

1½ pounds chicken livers, cleaned

3 tablespoons apple cider vinegar

In a large skillet, melt the ghee over medium heat. Add the garlic, onion, bay leaf, thyme, rosemary, and sage and season with the salt.

Add the livers and cook for 7 to 10 minutes.

Add the vinegar and cook for 3 to 5 minutes more.

Remove the herb stems and transfer the liver mixture to a blender or food processor. Blend until smooth. If you would like to thin the pâté, add some water (up to ½ cup).

Serve immediately, or transfer to an airtight container and refrigerate for up to 1 week. This also freezes really well! Scoop the pâté in tablespoon portions onto a parchment paper–lined baking sheet, freeze until solid, then transfer to a zip-top bag and return to the freezer for up to 6 months.

tip

NOT USED TO EATING LIVER PÂTÉ? TRY TO THINK OF IT LIKE YOU WOULD HUMMUS—AS A DELICIOUS DIP OR NUTRIENT-RICH SPREAD ON YOUR COLLARD WRAPS (PAGE 100) OR SANDWICH CREATIONS.

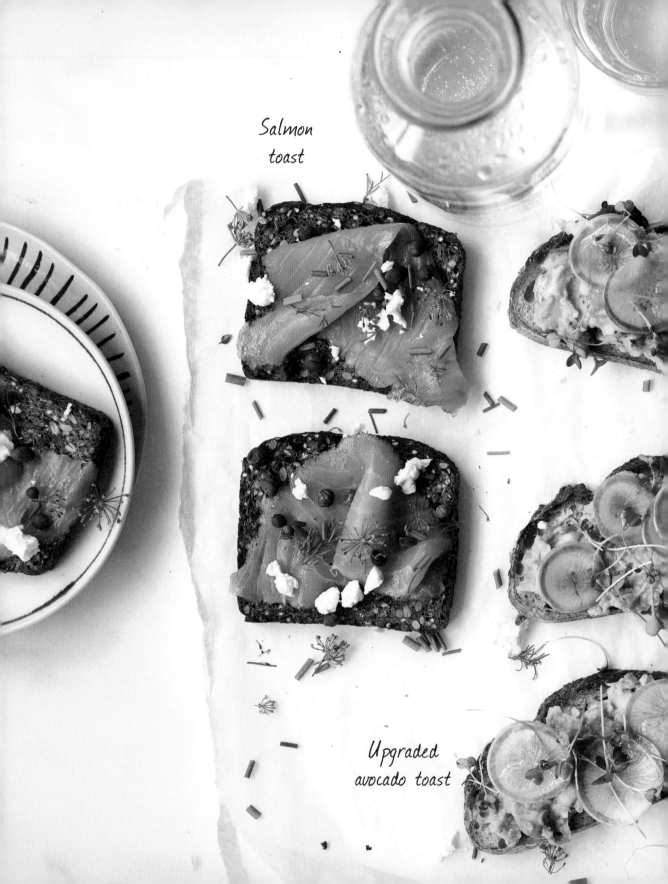

Salmon
toast

Upgraded
avocado toast

SHOW ME YOUR TOASTS

TURN THE PAGE FOR MY FAVORITE UPGRADED TOAST IDEAS!

Ricotta fig toast

◇

SHOW ME YOUR TOASTS

Do you remember life before avocado toast? What were we all eating (and photographing)?? There's a good reason it's so popular: toast is totally versatile and lends itself to easy meals that are also visually appealing. Think of a slice of toast as a blank canvas on which to express your creativity. Here are eight upgraded toast ideas, and I want you to show me your best slice. Snap a photo, post to social, and tag me @RobynYoukilis so I can see your creations!

Salmon Toast—Top your toast with smoked salmon, capers, chives, and crumbled goat cheese.

Upgraded Avocado Toast—Mash avocado and sauerkraut together, top with thinly sliced radishes, sprouts, salt and pepper, and a drizzle of extra-virgin olive oil.

Ricotta Fig Toast—Spread ricotta cheese on your toast and top with sliced figs and a drizzle of raw honey.

Sweet Potato Toast—Swap your bread for a slice of roasted sweet potato and top with almond butter, sliced pear, and a sprinkle of cinnamon.

Bone Marrow Toast—Spoon bone marrow on your toast and top with quick pickled onions and fresh herbs like thyme or parsley.

Beet Hummus Toast—Spread your toast with Beautiful Beet Hummus (page 148) and top with spicy microgreens.

Broccoli Toast—Chop up some Crispy Coconut Broccoli (page 156) and pile it on your toast. Garnish with lemon zest.

Liver Toast—Spread your toast with my Love Your Liver Pâté (page 149) and top with caramelized onions and snipped fresh chives.

Shroom Toast—Top your toast with sauteed mushrooms and chopped fresh parsley.

HONEYMOON GREENS

◇

While I love a giant plate of straight-up steamed greens drizzled with pumpkin seed oil and sea salt, sometimes my taste buds want something a little more complex. This variation of sautéed greens does the trick—the combination of ginger, lime, and shallots was inspired by my honeymoon in Bali, where these flavors were everywhere.

---

serves 2

2 to 3 tablespoons coconut
   or extra-virgin olive oil
1 bunch dark leafy greens, stemmed,
   leaves chopped and dried
2 or 3 shallots, minced or grated
1 (1½-inch) piece fresh ginger,
   peeled and grated
Sea salt and freshly ground black pepper
Fresh lime juice
Red pepper flakes (optional)

In a large sauté pan, melt 1 to 2 tablespoons of the oil over medium-low heat.

Add the greens, shallots, and ginger, season generously with salt and pepper, and mix well.

Cook, stirring, for 5 to 8 minutes, until the greens are softened and darken in color.

Drizzle the remaining 1 tablespoon olive or coconut oil over the greens and stir through. Scoop the greens from the pan onto two plates and serve with a squeeze of lime and a sprinkle of red pepper flakes, if desired.

$\diamond$

SOCCA FLATBREAD

I love getting my creative juices flowing in the kitchen, but even after all my years behind the stove, I'm still not much of a baker. For this reason I turn to quick breads and no-fuss flatbread recipes, like this socca. If you've discovered that gluten isn't your best friend, or are just looking for an easy starch to complete a meal, this flatbread is for you.

---

makes 1 thick or 2 thin 10-inch flatbreads

1 cup chickpea flour (also labeled gram flour or besan)

1 teaspoon sea salt

2 teaspoons olive oil, plus more for drizzling

VARIATIONS

Garlic Leek: ½ cup chopped leek, sautéed in oil or butter; 1 tablespoon garlic powder

Cheezy Rosemary: 1 tablespoon nutritional yeast, 1 tablespoon chopped fresh rosemary

Cinnamon Raisin: ¼ cup raisins, 1 teaspoon ground cinnamon

tip

POUR A THIN LAYER OF THE BATTER INTO EACH WELL OF A SILICONE MUFFIN PAN AND BAKE AS DIRECTED TO MAKE SOCCA "CRACKERS."

Preheat the oven to 425°F.

Combine the chickpea flour, sea salt, olive oil, and 1 cup water in a bowl, stir, and let sit for 30 minutes. Place a large cast-iron skillet in the oven to warm up for 10 minutes.

Add an additional drizzle of olive oil to the batter, then stir in the ingredients for the variation of your choice.

Add a drizzle of olive oil to your pan before adding the socca mixture. If making two thin flatbreads, carefully pour half the batter into the hot cast-iron pan in the oven. If making one thick flatbread, pour all the batter into the pan.

Bake for 10 to 15 minutes, until the edges begin to brown. Repeat to make a second thin pancake, if needed.

Use a spatula to remove the flatbread from the skillet. Slice and serve. You can enjoy as is or use like gluten-free pizza crust.

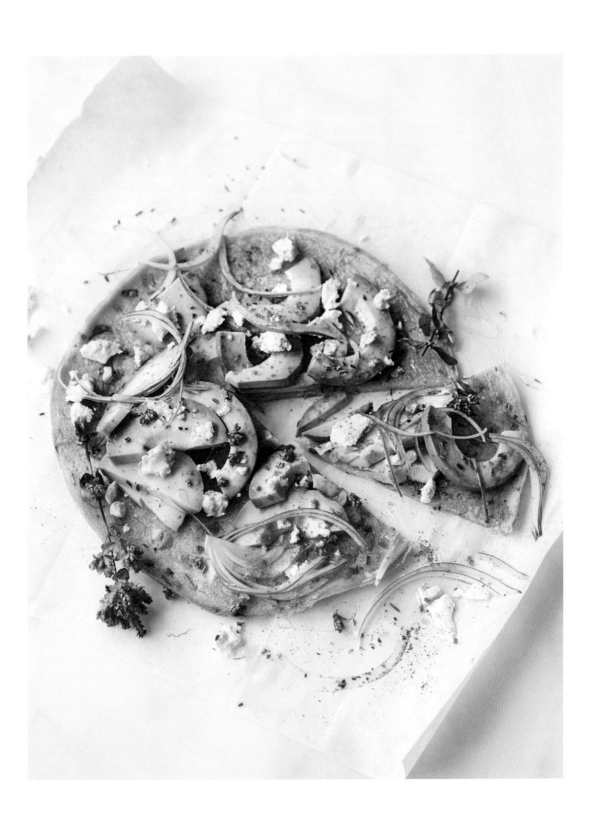

CRISPY COCONUT BROCCOLI

Toasty, crispy broccoli was a classic go-to my mom made for our family and guests. Even the people who said they didn't like broccoli always loved this version. I made a few swaps to my mom's recipe, like adding in shredded coconut for a dose of healthy fats and fiber. It makes a great side dish for any weeknight dinner or company meal.

serves 3 or a 4 as a side

3 heads broccoli, chopped into florets
1 tablespoon coconut oil, melted (see Tip)
Sea salt and freshly ground black pepper
3 tablespoons unsweetened coconut flakes

Preheat the oven to 425°F.

Toss the broccoli with the coconut oil, spread on a baking sheet in a single layer, and season with salt and pepper.

Bake for 25 minutes. Remove the baking sheet from the oven and sprinkle the coconut flakes over the broccoli.

Bake for 5 minutes more, or until the coconut is lightly toasted. Serve hot.

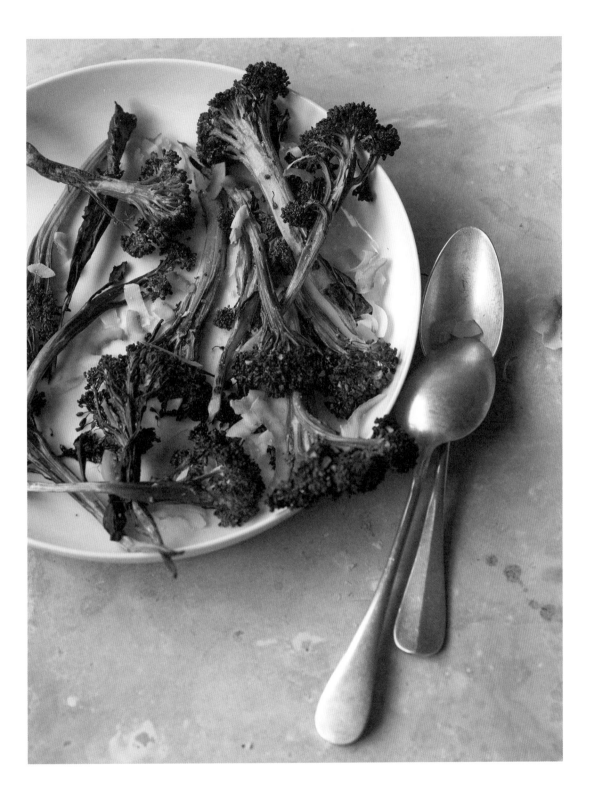

HERBED QUINOA PILAF

◇

I love how quinoa has its own nutty flavor, but is also enough of a blank slate to add any veggies, herbs, sauces, and proteins too. Most of my recipes call for lots of herbs, and this quinoa is one easy way to use up leftovers. Make a big batch at the beginning of the week and enjoy it with your lunch or dinner.

serves 6

3½ cups water or broth or a mix of the two

2 cups quinoa

2 teaspoons sea salt

Leaves from 1 sprig rosemary, coarsely chopped

2 fresh sage leaves, finely chopped

Leaves from 3 to 5 sprigs thyme

1 tablespoon ghee, coconut, or olive oil

In a medium saucepan, bring the water or broth to a boil. Add the quinoa, salt, rosemary, sage, thyme, and ghee or oil and stir. Reduce the heat to low, cover, and simmer until the quinoa is cooked through and fluffy, about 20 minutes.

Remove from the heat. Fluff with a fork and serve.

◇

GOOD GUT GREEN RICE

This green rice is an easy go-to grain, and it pairs well with almost all my protein and veggie recipes. You can add a sauce if you want to get fancy, but it's also delicious as is.

serves 6

2 cups white rice
  (basmati or jasmine work well)
1 tablespoon ghee or coconut oil
1 leek, white and light green parts,
  thinly sliced and washed well
1 to 2 teaspoons sea salt
Freshly ground black pepper
Leaves from ½ bunch parsley, chopped
Leaves from ½ bunch cilantro, chopped

Rinse the rice in a fine-mesh strainer.

In a large pot, melt the ghee over medium heat. Add the leek, season with the salt and pepper, and cook, stirring, until softened, 5 to 7 minutes.

Add the rice and toast for about 1 minute.

Add 3 cups water, raise the heat to medium-high, and bring to a boil.

Reduce the heat to low, cover, and cook until the rice is tender but not mushy, about 20 minutes.

Fluff with a fork, stir in the parsley and cilantro, and cover for 5 minutes more before serving.

ARTICHOKE-STYLE BRUSSELS SPROUTS

◇

You heard it from me first: Brussels sprouts chips are the new kale chips. When I tested this recipe, I had some leftover aioli in the fridge, and BOOM the most amazing flavor combination was born. Try this recipe for a fancy (but easy) twist on basic roasted veggies.

serves 6

1½ pounds Brussels sprouts, trimmed and halved

3 tablespoons avocado or olive oil

1 teaspoon sea salt

Freshly ground black pepper

AIOLI

½ cup mayonnaise (I use the kinds made out of avocado and olive oils)

1 garlic clove, minced

½ teaspoon lemon zest

2 teaspoons fresh lemon juice

Pinch of sea salt

1 teaspoon fresh thyme

Pinch of red pepper flakes (optional)

Preheat the oven to 400°F.

Toss the Brussels sprouts with the olive oil, salt, and pepper to taste and place on a baking sheet. Bake for 35 to 45 minutes, until browned and crispy.

Meanwhile, mix all the aioli ingredients together in a small bowl and set aside until the Brussels sprouts are ready to enjoy.

note

THIS RECIPE CALLS FOR MAYONNAISE. YOU'LL WANT TO REACH FOR A VERSION MADE WITHOUT SOYBEAN OR CANOLA OIL, OR CHALLENGE YOURSELF TO MAKE YOUR OWN. THE AIOLI IS ALSO DELICIOUS WITH THE 'BOOCH-BATTERED FISH AND CHIPS (PAGE 131).

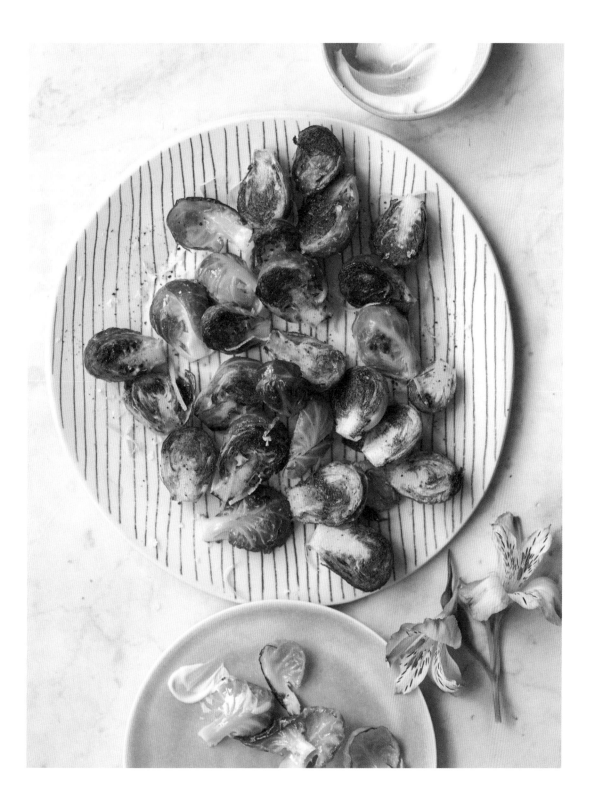

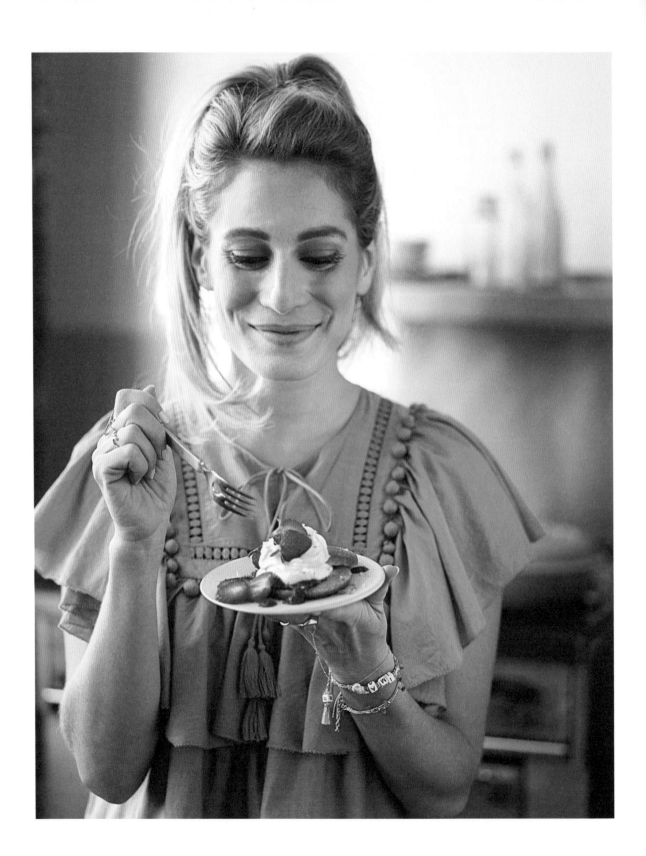

SWEET TREATS

FABULOUS FRUIT SALAD

The key to this unusual fruit salad is the combination of fresh and dried fruit. It's perfect for parties and potlucks, because let's be honest: Everyone loves the person who brings a beautiful fruit salad. Bonus: the leftovers (if there are any!) are delicious in my Power Parfait (page 36).

serves 4

2 seedless oranges, peeled, sectioned,
   and cut into halves
Seeds from 1 pomegranate, or about 1 cup
   ready-to-serve pomegranate seeds
2 pears, cored and thinly sliced lengthwise
1 apple, cored and thinly sliced
¾ cup mix of dried apricots and Turkish
   figs, chopped
2 teaspoons raw honey
Juice of 1 lemon
Handful of fresh mint leaves, chopped

Combine the fresh and dried fruits in a bowl.

Drizzle with the honey and lemon juice, add the mint, and mix together.

Let sit to macerate for at least 20 minutes before serving.

◇

GOOD-GUT GELLIES

After having my daughter, I couldn't seem to GO in the morning. What finally worked were these by-accident apple juice jellies that came together when I left my apple juice and psyllium husk mixture sitting on the counter and it thickened up. My herbalist recommended this combo, and it's the only thing that got me going. On days I ate these, I went, and on days I didn't—I didn't. If you're struggling to get regular, try these ASAP.

---

serves 2

½ cup organic apple juice or cider
  (try to get the most natural version you
  can with no added sugar)
2 tablespoons whole psyllium husk
Sprinkle of cinnamon (optional)

In a small jar or container, mix together the apple juice, psyllium, and cinnamon, if using.

Refrigerate to firm up for at least 15 minutes or up to overnight. Enjoy!

tip

PSYLLIUM HUSK IS PURE SOLUBLE FIBER AND PROMOTES EASY ELIMINATION BY PULLING WASTE OUT OF THE COLON MORE QUICKLY AND EFFICIENTLY. IT'S ALSO A PREBIOTIC FOOD, WHICH MAKES IT A GO WITH YOUR GUT FAVORITE!

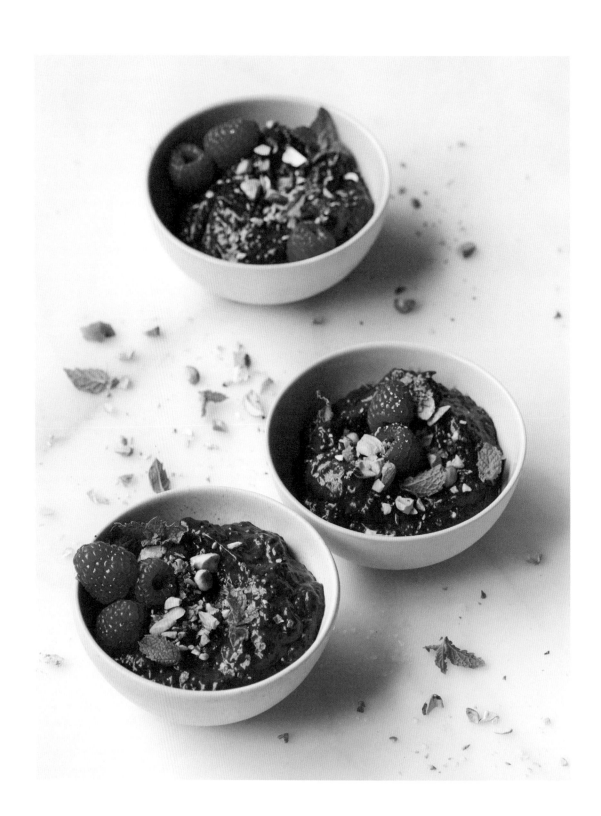

$\Diamond$

SALTED DARK CHOCOLATE PUDDING

Sometimes we just need chocolate, and this pudding is a great treat when a square of dark chocolate won't do the job. You can't taste the avocado in here, but it makes this pudding rich and creamy. The fiber from the avocado, chia seeds, and cacao will help stabilize your blood sugar, so there's no crash that's common with so many sugar-laden desserts. Bonus: Kids love it, too!

serves 2

1 ripe avocado, pitted and peeled

⅔ cup milk of choice

2 tablespoons chia seeds

¼ cup raw cacao powder
  or unsweetened cocoa powder

2 tablespoons date syrup
  (can swap for maple syrup)

¼ teaspoon sea salt,
  plus more for garnish if desired

1 teaspoon pure vanilla extract

Fresh mint, raspberries,
  and toasted nuts, for garnish

Combine all the ingredients in a blender or food processor and blend until smooth.

Finish with a sprinkle of sea salt and garnish with fresh mint, raspberries, and toasted nuts.

◇

CHAI GINGERBREAD COOKIES

I love gingerbread cookies, but despite the fact that they contain digestion-friendly ginger, most traditional recipes have tons of white sugar and white flour. So instead of having to pass altogether, I made some swaps and came up with this Robyn-approved version that's almost as healthy as a breakfast cookie (for a real cookie you can eat for breakfast, head to page 76). These cookies also contain turmeric, which is anti-inflammatory and great for your entire bod.

---

makes about 16 cookies

6 tablespoons coconut oil,
   plus more for greasing

1 teaspoon pure vanilla extract

¼ cup molasses

2 cups oat flour

¼ cup coconut sugar

2 teaspoons baking powder

1 teaspoon baking soda

2 teaspoons grated fresh ginger

1 teaspoon grated fresh turmeric

1 teaspoon ground cinnamon

½ teaspoon ground cardamom

Pinch of sea salt

Freshly ground black pepper

¼ cup coconut milk
   or nondairy milk of choice

¼ cup chopped crystallized ginger (optional)

Preheat the oven to 350°F. Line a baking sheet with parchment paper or grease it with oil.

In a small saucepan, melt the coconut oil over medium heat. Add the vanilla and molasses and stir to combine.

In a large bowl, combine the flour, sugar, baking powder, baking soda, fresh ginger, turmeric, cinnamon, cardamom, salt, and pepper to taste. Stir to combine.

Add the melted coconut oil mixture to the bowl and mix to incorporate. Add the coconut milk and mix together. If using crystallized ginger, gently fold it into the dough.

The batter will be sticky—you can place it in the freezer for 15 minutes so that it will be easier to work with. Use your hands to form batter into 2-inch balls. Place the balls on a baking sheet about 1½ inches apart and flatten lightly with your palm. Bake for 8 to 12 minutes, or until the edges are browned and crispy. Store the cookies in an airtight container at room temperature for up to 1 week. These also freeze well!

◇

MOM'S HONEY CAKE-ISH

This recipe was a happy accident: I was working on a veggie-packed muffin for this book and ended up with a variation that tasted almost like my mom's Passover honey cake, which is out of this world delicious. I still can't believe how good this recipe tastes, considering that it's almost all veggies and sweetened with just a teeny ¼ cup of raw honey.

makes about 8 muffins

Coconut oil spray

¾ cup grated zucchini

¾ cup grated carrots

2 large eggs

2 tablespoons coconut oil, melted

½ teaspoon pure vanilla extract

¼ cup raw honey

1 cup almond flour

1 teaspoon ground cinnamon

½ teaspoon baking soda

½ teaspoon baking powder

Pinch of sea salt

Preheat the oven to 350°F. Grease eight wells of a standard muffin tin with coconut oil spray.

Combine the zucchini and carrots in a large bowl. Add the eggs, coconut oil, vanilla, and honey and mix well.

In a medium bowl, mix together the almond flour, cinnamon, baking soda, baking powder, and salt.

Slowly add the flour mixture to the veggie mixture and mix until combined.

Divide the batter evenly among the prepared wells of the muffin tin and bake for 20 to 25 minutes, until golden brown.

Cool and then store in the fridge, loosely covered, for up to 5 days.

◇
STRAWBERRY SHORTCAKES

Strawberry shortcake is my favorite dessert in the world, so I made a healthy version I can eat more often than the real deal. This is actually three awesome recipes in one: You can use the cakes as breakfast biscuits, the frosting on healthy cupcakes, and the strawberry chia jam on toast or yogurt!

---

makes 12 mini cakes

CAKES

¾ cup coconut oil, melted

6 large eggs

1½ teaspoons pure vanilla extract

⅓ cup coconut sugar or pure maple syrup

¾ cup coconut flour

½ teaspoon sea salt

½ teaspoon baking soda

JAM

1 cup strawberries, chopped

1 tablespoon fresh lemon juice

1 tablespoon raw honey

2 tablespoons chia seeds

FROSTING

2 (14-ounce) cans coconut milk,
   refrigerated overnight

¼ cup raw honey

1 teaspoon pure vanilla extract

Pinch of sea salt

GARNISHES

½ cup sliced fresh strawberries

Fresh mint leaves

Make the cakes: Preheat the oven to 350°F. Grease a muffin tin with a little of the coconut oil (or use coconut oil spray). In a large bowl, combine the eggs, vanilla, the remaining coconut oil, and the coconut sugar. Slowly add the flour, salt, and baking soda. Whisk to combine. Pour into the tin and bake for 25 to 30 minutes, until golden and firm on top.

Make the jam: In a saucepan over medium heat, combine the strawberries and ¼ cup water and cook until falling apart. Add the lemon juice and honey and cook, stirring with whisk occasionally, for 5 minutes more. Remove from the heat and stir in the chia seeds. Let sit for at least 10 minutes before serving.

Make the frosting: Open the cans of coconut milk and pour off the clear liquid. Put the thick coconut cream in a medium bowl, add the honey, vanilla, and salt, and whisk until smooth.

Assemble and garnish the cakes: Let the cakes cool completely in the muffin tins, then turn them out onto a plate or platter. Slice in half.

Spread the chia jam over the bottom half of the cake. Add a large dollop of frosting and stack the second half of the cake on top. Repeat with remaining cakes. Garnish with additional frosting, sliced strawberries, and mint leaves. Serve and eat immediately.

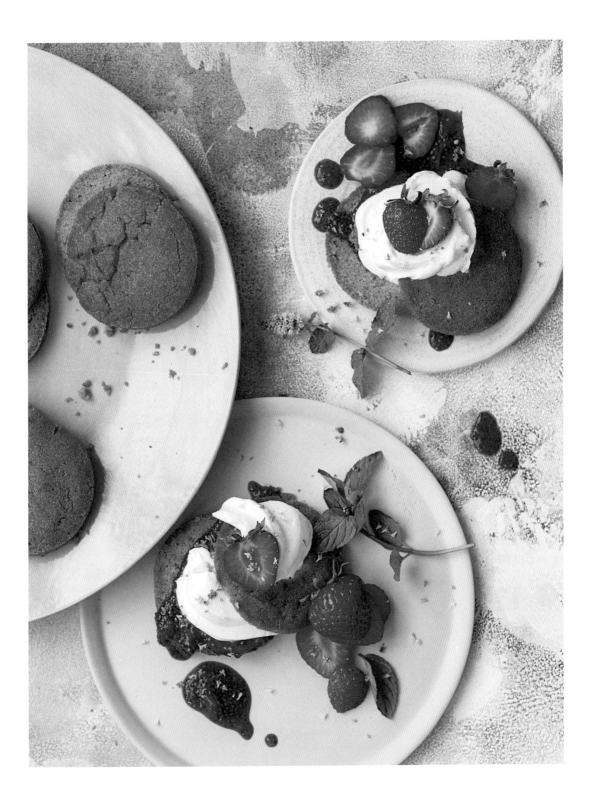

◇

GOOD-GUT DELIGHT

I was always fascinated by Turkish delight as a kid—I thought it was the coolest dessert. I don't even know if I liked the flavor, I just thought it was so unique and pretty. Now as an adult, I love these upgraded gelatin gummies inspired by the flavors of traditional Turkish delight. Gelatin helps heal the gut lining, and rose water is calming for your belly, making these the perfect afternoon snack or evening sweet treat.

---

serving size depends on shape and cut

⅓ cup pure pomegranate juice

¼ cup raw honey

¼ cup powdered grass-fed gelatin

1 tablespoon rose water

¼ cup chopped pistachios (optional)

2 to 3 tablespoons arrowroot powder, for dusting (optional)

In a saucepan, combine the pomegranate juice, honey, and 2 cups water. Heat over medium heat until simmering.

In a small bowl, whisk the gelatin into ½ cup water and set aside for 5 minutes.

Stir the rose water into the pomegranate juice mixture. Add the gelatin mixture and stir well until the gelatin is dissolved. Remove from the heat and add the pistachios (if using).

Line an 8-by-8-inch glass baking dish with parchment paper, leaving about 1 inch of overhang on all sides. Pour the mixture into the dish, cover, and refrigerate for at least 3 hours or up to overnight. Once the gelatin has set, cut it into rectangles or the size and shape of your choice.

Put the arrowroot powder in a pie plate or deep dish. Dust the gummies in the arrowroot to coat before serving. You can also drizzle them with melted chocolate!

Store in an airtight container in the fridge for up to 10 days.

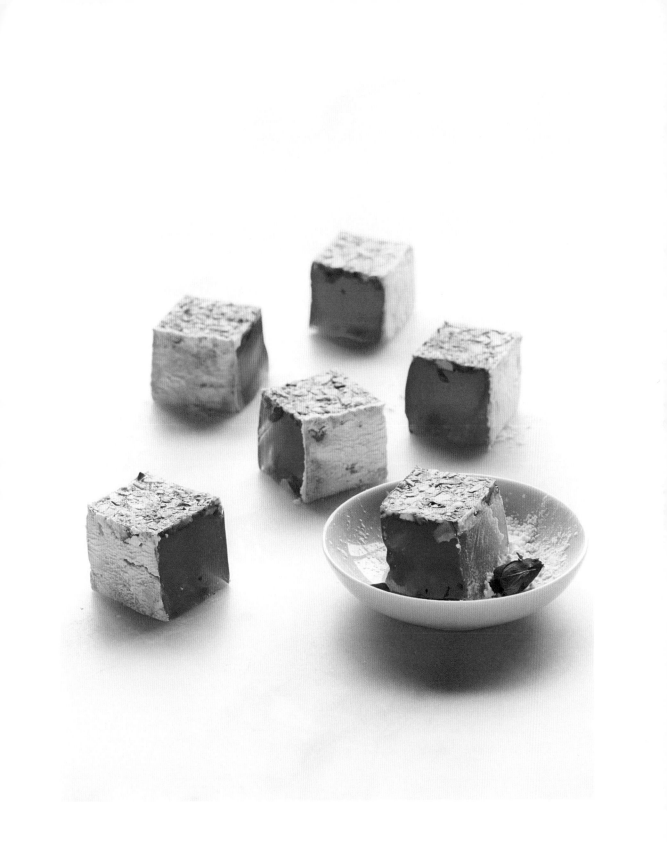

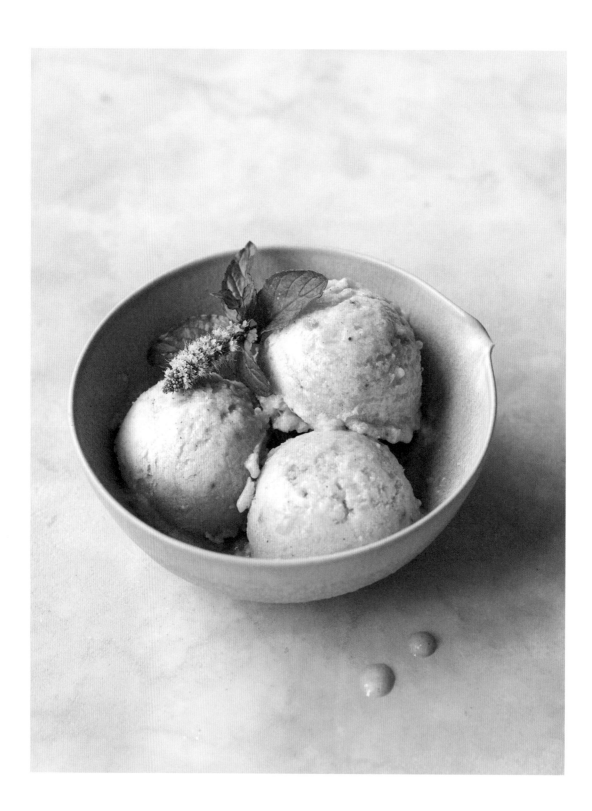

PEACHES 'N CREAM NICE CREAM

◇

"Nice cream" is a standard warm weather dessert in my household. I came up with this variation to highlight my daughter, Navy's, favorite summertime fruit: Peaches! The addition of coconut milk and frozen banana adds the perfect amount of creaminess to the peaches. Can't find peaches? This recipe works with any frozen fruit.

serves 2

2 cups frozen peaches

½ frozen ripe banana

¼ cup full-fat coconut milk

½ teaspoon vanilla extract

Dash of cinnamon

1 small scoop collagen protein (optional)

Fresh mint, for garnish (optional)

Add all the ingredients except the mint to a high-speed blender or food processor. Blend until smooth (you may need to pulse a few times and scrape down the sides).

Divide into two small bowls, garnish with the mint if you like, and enjoy immediately!

note

YOU CAN ALSO MAKE THIS NICE CREAM "SCOOPABLE." DOUBLE THE RECIPE AND POUR INTO A STANDARD LOAF PAN LINED WITH PARCHMENT PAPER. FREEZE FOR AT LEAST 2 TO 3 HOURS OR OVERNIGHT SO IT HARDENS ENOUGH TO SCOOP WITH AN ICE CREAM SCOOPER.

◇

SECRET TRUFFLES

Okay, don't immediately turn the page when you see the first ingredient here—I promise these truffles do not taste a thing like beans! When blended well, black beans have a creamy texture that makes them a nice base for healthy truffles. When I have good chocolate around, I'll eat most of the bar in one sitting. With these truffles, I am able to have just two or three perfect bites and be good to go.

---

makes 10 to 15 truffles

TRUFFLES

1 (15-ounce) can black beans, drained and rinsed very well

2 tablespoons pure maple syrup

3 tablespoons coconut oil

3 tablespoons unsweetened cocoa powder

2 tablespoons coconut butter

½ teaspoon pure vanilla extract

Pinch of sea salt

OPTIONAL TOPPINGS:

Crushed pistachios

Unsweetened coconut flakes

Unsweetened cocoa powder

Sea salt

Toasted sesame seeds

Cayenne pepper

Combine all the truffle ingredients in a blender or food processor and blend until smooth.

Form truffles by rolling about 2 tablespoons of the bean mixture into balls with your hands and set them on a plate.

Roll the truffles in your favorite toppings!

Refrigerate for at least 30 minutes before serving. Store in the fridge in an airtight container for up to 1 week, or in the freezer for up to 1 month.

tip

YOU CAN EXPERIMENT WITH ADDING THE TOPPINGS DIRECTLY INTO THE TRUFFLE MIXTURE BASE TOO!

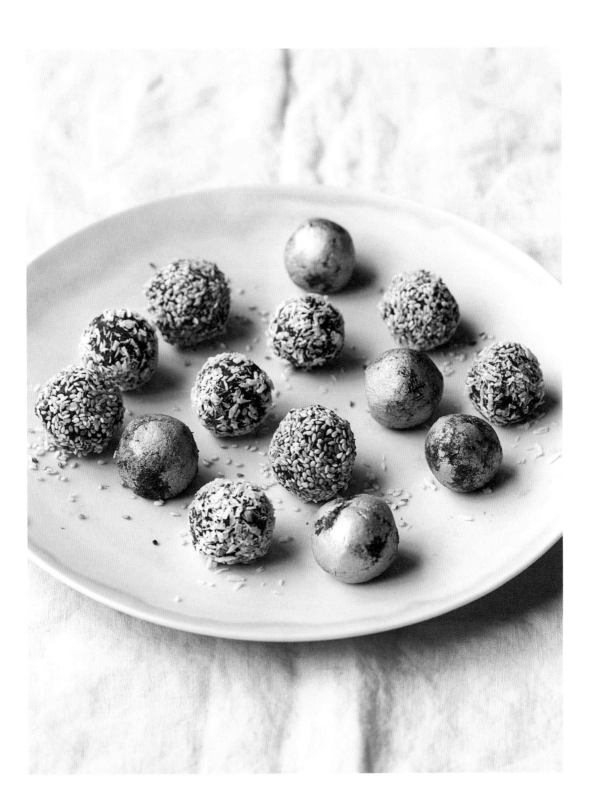

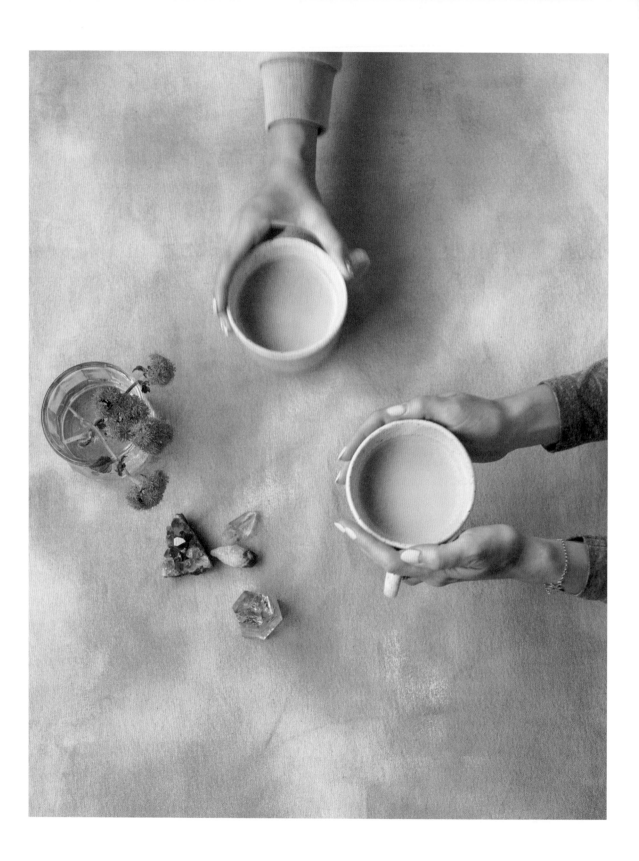

◇

DRINKS

———————

◇

GO WITH YOUR GUT LEMONADE

Back in the 90s, my mom was a Crystal Light lemonade queen, and truthfully, I loved it, too. This low-glycemic, gut-friendly version is a refreshing alternative to both the Crystal Light of my youth and today's sugar- or agave-loaded options. The cucumber and mint are soothing for your digestive system, and the fennel gives this drink a fun flavor twist.

---

serves 1

½ *small bulb fennel*

1 *lemon, peeled*

1 *Persian cucumber*

   (or ½ larger cucumber, peeled)

Handful of fresh mint leaves

Liquid stevia (optional)

Combine the fennel, lemon, cucumber, mint, and 2 cups cold water in a high-speed blender and blend for 30 seconds.

Pour through a fine-mesh strainer.

Taste and add more water or a drop or two of stevia, if desired.

fun variations

TRY USING SPARKLING WATER OR KOMBUCHA IN PLACE OF THE WATER. YOU CAN ALSO USE A JUICER (INSTEAD OF THE BLEND-AND-STRAIN PROCESS). IF YOU MAKE IT THIS WAY, TRY ADDING AN APPLE OR PEAR INSTEAD OF THE WATER AND OPTIONAL STEVIA.

FERMENTED FRUIT SODA

Kombucha is so last year . . . just kidding! But if you're looking for another cold, sweet, and bubbly beverage to add to your gut-friendly toolkit, you'll want to try this easy-peasy ferment. Traditionally known as fruit kvass, this "soda" is packed with good-for-your-gut probiotics and makes a great swap for traditional soda. Plus, kiddos of all ages love it.

makes about 4 cups

Ripe fruit of choice (see Note)

1 tablespoon raw honey

Filtered water

note

I TYPICALLY USE A MIX OF RASPBERRIES AND BLACKBERRIES BECAUSE THOSE ARE MY (AND NAVY'S) FAVORITES, BUT FEEL FREE TO EXPERIMENT WITH ANYTHING THAT'S IN SEASON. USE ENOUGH FRUIT TO FILL THE JAR BY ONE-THIRD TO ONE-HALF.

Place the fruit in a 2-quart mason jar.

Mix the honey with a small amount of warm filtered water so it slightly dissolves and becomes less viscous.

Add the honey mixture to the jar and cover with filtered water, leaving some room at the top of the jar. Stir and seal tightly.

Set aside in a cool, dark place to ferment for 2 to 3 days, shaking the jar twice daily to prevent bacteria from forming on the surface. After 24 hours, you should see fermentation bubbles! Taste your brew every day until you get that perfect mix of sweet and tangy that tastes best to you.

Strain the fruit soda (you can add the strained fruit to a smoothie for a probiotic fiber boost!), transfer to a clean jar, and store in the fridge for up to 2 weeks. You can drink it straight (start small, like 2 ounces) or add a tablespoon or two to your water throughout the day.

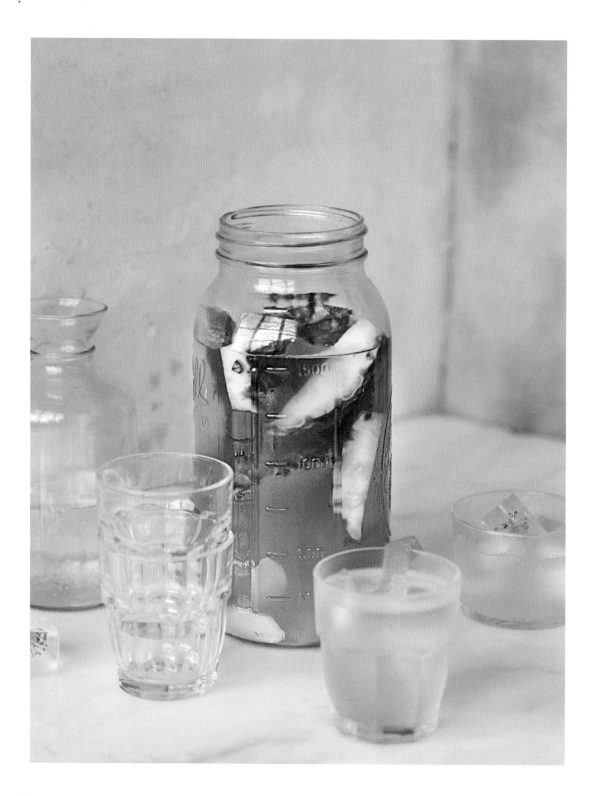

PINEAPPLE TEPACHE

Hot summer days and nights call for cooling beverages—and if they can be of the fermented variety, even better! Pineapple tepache is essentially a fermented agua fresca popular in Mexico and South America. This drink is lovely on its own but also makes a special base for upgraded cocktails (and mocktails!).

makes about 8 cups

1 pineapple

½ to 1 cup sweetener of choice
   (coconut sugar works great!)

1 (1-inch) piece fresh ginger,
   peeled and sliced

Filtered water

tip

MY FAVORITE WAY TO ENJOY THIS DRINK IS TO USE IT TO FLAVOR PLAIN SPARKLING WATER (ABOUT A 1-TO-3 RATIO OF TEPACHE TO WATER).

Rinse the pineapple lightly with water. You want to keep some of the natural yeasts that start the fermentation process. Cut the crown from the pineapple, then thickly cut off the peel so there is ¼ to ½ inch of fruit left on the peel. Set the fruit without the peel aside to enjoy another time.

If you are using a granulated sweetener, first dissolve it in a small amount of hot water.

Place the pineapple peels and ginger in the bottom of a 2-quart jar. Add the sweetener to the jar and add filtered water to cover.

Weigh down the peels (you can do this with the crown of the pineapple) and cover the jar with a dishtowel or cheesecloth. Use a rubber band to secure the cover. Set aside in a cool, dark place to ferment for 1 to 5 days, checking the flavor daily to achieve desired taste. The longer you ferment, the sourer and fizzier it will be.

When the tepache is fermented to your liking, train it, and serve over ice or store in a clean jar in the fridge.

◇

MAGICAL MORNING MATCHA

This loaded matcha latte is deliciously frothy and gives a noticeable energy boost without the jitters and funky gut flare-ups that sometimes accompany drinking regular coffee. Plus, it's a sweet vehicle for your current favorite superfoods and adaptogens—and looks great on your social feed. Try this recipe, then post your Magical Morning Matcha to Instagram and tag me @RobynYoukilis and #YourHealthiestYou.

serves 1

1 teaspoon ceremonial grade
   matcha powder
2 cups water, homemade hemp milk,
   or a mix of the two
1 tablespoon coconut butter (can swap for
   ghee, but it will be a little less frothy)
1 to 2 scoops collagen powder
¼ to ½ teaspoon medicinal herbs, such as
   ashwagandha, rhodiola, or maca
   (I suggest no more than two at a time)

Bring the water to a near boil or bring the hemp milk (or hemp milk–water mixture) to a simmer in a small saucepan. Set aside to cool slightly, 3 to 5 minutes.

Combine the remaining ingredients in a blender.

Add the water or hemp milk (or the mixture) to the blender and blend for up to 1 minute.

Taste and adjust the ingredients if needed.

Pour, sip, and enjoy!

tip

FOR EASY HOMEMADE HEMP MILK,
BLEND 3 TABLESPOONS HEMP SEEDS
AND 4 CUPS WATER

◇

THREE-SEED
TEA

This traditional Ayurvedic tea is great for reducing bloating and inflammation in your digestive system. The combination of these three potent spices makes a healing tonic that's naturally caffeine-free so you can enjoy this soothing cup any time of day or night.

---

serves 5 or 6

1 teaspoon cumin seeds

1 teaspoon coriander seeds

1 teaspoon fennel seeds

Squeeze of fresh lemon or lime juice
  (optional)

Bring 5 to 6 cups water to a boil in a medium saucepan. Add the seeds and reduce the heat to maintain a simmer.

Simmer for 5 to 10 minutes, depending on how strong you want the flavor.

Cool, then strain through a fine-mesh strainer into a glass jar or bottle. Add the lemon or lime juice, if using.

Drink 1 cup immediately and refrigerate the rest for later.

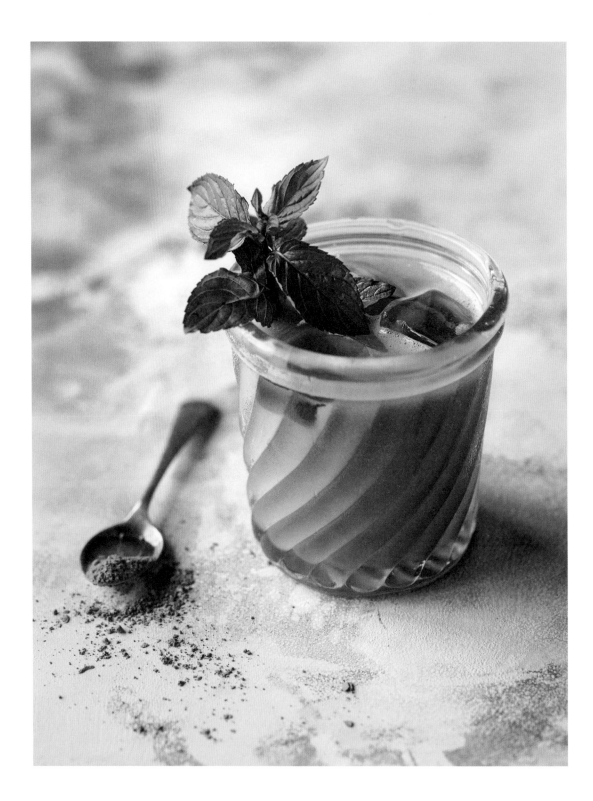

◇

CHOCO-MINT MATCHA LATTE

I discovered a rooftop herb garden on my building one evening while chasing a view of the sunset. And OMG, they had chocolate mint! Yep, it's a real thing. The herb works perfectly here, as it naturally lightens up traditionally earthy matcha in this fun variation of an iced tea latte. No chocolate mint? No problem. Regular mint and 1 teaspoon unsweetened cocoa powder will work just fine!

---

serves 1

½ cup unsweetened vanilla milk alternative
  (I like almond or coconut here)
1 teaspoon ceremonial grade
  matcha powder
Small handful of fresh chocolate
  mint leaves

tip

YOU CAN PURCHASE A HIGH-QUALITY "INSTANT" STYLE MATCHA THAT'S MEANT TO MIX DIRECTLY INTO COLD LIQUIDS. IF YOU'VE GOT THIS TYPE OF MATCHA, YOU CAN SIMPLY ADD ALL OF THE INGREDIENTS STRAIGHT INTO THE MASON JAR, SEAL, AND SHAKE (AND SKIP THE WHOLE FIRST STEP).

Heat the milk alternative in a small saucepan to a low simmer. Whisk in the matcha vigorously or blend in a high-speed blender.

Add the milk mixture, 1 cup of cold water, the mint leaves, and a handful of ice cubes to a large mason jar with a lid.

Seal and shake until well combined.

Add more ice cubes if needed, strain the mint, and enjoy!

◇

KOMBUCHA COCKTAIL

The first bitters were created purely for medicinal purposes to help cure seasickness and stomach ailments. This cocktail incorporates digestion-friendly bitters and probiotic-rich kombucha for a fun and healthy elixir. This cocktail is equally fabulous with or without the booze. Cheers!

---

serves 1

Ice

1 tablespoon fresh ginger juice

Juice of ½ lime

Juice of ½ lemon

1 shot vodka (or additional kombucha if
   making a mocktail version)

5 dashes of bitters

½ cup kombucha

Slice of lemon or lime peel, for garnish
   (optional)

Fill half of a cocktail shaker (or large mason jar with lid) with ice. Add the ginger, lime, lemon, vodka, and bitters and shake well.

Put the kombucha in a tall glass. Strain the vodka mixture over the kombucha. Stir well and garnish with a twist.

tip

YOU CAN MAKE GINGER JUICE WITHOUT A JUICER! SIMPLY GRATE FRESH GINGER ROOT ON A MICROPLANE GRATER AND SQUEEZE THE PULP TO EXTRACT THE JUICE.

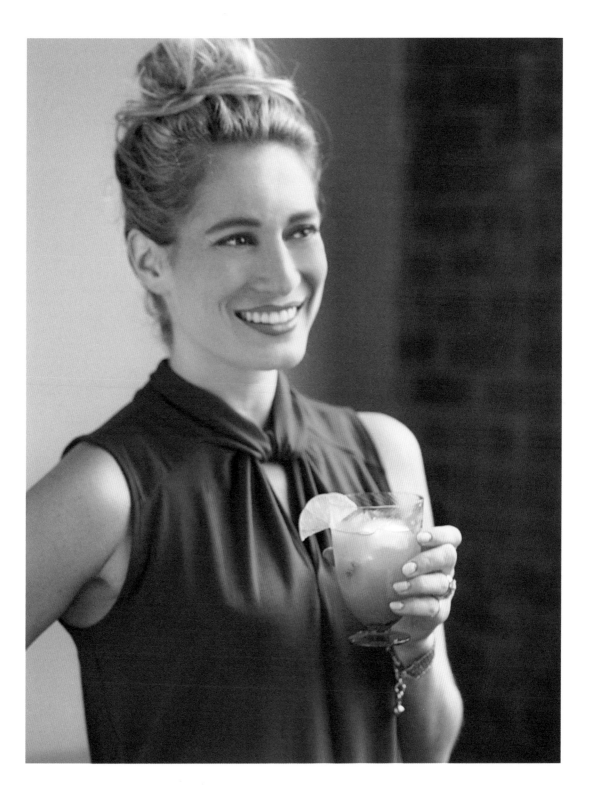

INDEX

THANK YOU!

From the bottom of my heart, thank you to every client, friend, teacher, and moment of inspiration that made this book all that it is. To my book team, especially Kyle, Ellen, Nicky, and Gaby, for seeing my vision and bringing it to life. To my editor, Chris, for your hard work, humor, and flexibility with my usually missed deadlines. Thank you to my fabulous literary agents, Sarah and Celeste. Thank you Emily for your dedication and for making my work fun again. To my family, my nearest and dearest, especially my mama and brother. To my daughter, Navy, for giving me the gift of you, and the gift of finally feeling at peace in my body. And to my husband, Scott, thank you for supporting me body, mind, and soul through this process. For stepping into our next level of us, and for reminding me that you like my tush, just the way it is.